中醫舌診

Tongue Diagnosis in Chinese Medicine

REVISED EDITION

Giovanni Maciocia

Eastland Press
SEATTLE

Library of Congress Catalog Card Number: 94-61961
International Standard Book Number: 0-939616-19-X
Printed in the United States of America.

Book design by Catherine L. Nelson.
Brush calligraphy by Kou Hoi-Yin.

The French and Dutch language editions of this book
are published by SATAS (Belgium), the German edition
by ML Verlag (Germany), and the Hungarian edition
by Les Editions 3•8•3 Publishing Ltd. (Hungary).

To My Wife

Table of Contents

Preface to Revised Edition

Tongue diagnosis is one of the most precious diagnostic methods in Chinese medicine. Its basic elements are relatively easy to learn, but like many aspects of Chinese medicine, it is constantly enriched by clinical practice. No matter how long one has been practicing, there will always be something new to learn. In fact, in every lecture I give on tongue diagnosis there is always at least one student who describes a type of tongue that I have never seen before!

The beauty of tongue diagnosis lies in its simplicity and immediacy: whenever there is a complex disorder full of contradictions, examination of the tongue instantly clarifies the main pathological process. In the past few years I have also found tongue diagnosis to be an invaluable tool for discerning a strong emotional aspect in the condition of a patient, for discriminating between the principal and secondary aspects of a complex disorder, and for choosing the appropriate method of treatment in herbal therapy.

New and expanded subjects discussed in this revised edition of *Tongue Diagnosis in Chinese Medicine* include:

- Western anatomy of the tongue
- Tongue diagnosis in children
- Tongue diagnosis and herbal therapy
- Clinical significance of tongue diagnosis in complex disorders
- The effect of drugs on the tongue
- New case histories and color plates of tongues

The reader's attention is especially directed to the new chapter on the clinical significance of tongue diagnosis. This chapter contains a number of guidelines for the interpretation of the tongue in complex disorders, the use of tongue diagnosis in discerning emotional problems, and the integration of tongue and pulse diagnosis.

Although it could be argued that tongue diagnosis is more important for herbalists than it is for acupuncturists, I personally believe that the conditions of practice in the West are different than those in China, where the specialties of acupuncture and herbal medicine are fairly rigidly separated. During my visits to China I met very few doctors who practiced both acupuncture and herbal medicine; in fact, only two come to mind. In the West, however, we have been cast in the role of "alternative" primary health care providers, much like general practitioners. Patients do not come looking only for the "channel work" typical of acupuncture, but want to know why they are ill, what influence diet has on their condition, and the nature of their diagnosis (in Chinese terms) and prognosis. Tongue diagnosis provides invaluable information for all of these aspects of clinical practice, whether we use acupuncture or herbs.

Yet another advantage of tongue diagnosis is its value in self-diagnosis. After a patient has been to the clinic a few times, he or she is often intrigued by tongue diagnosis and will begin to examine their own tongue on a daily basis. Occasionally, patients who were previously discharged return later when they notice the appearance of a thick coating or a particular swelling on the tongue. This common fascination with tongue diagnosis contributes to greater patient involvement in the early detection and treatment of a condition.

Finally, a few words about the translation and capitalization of Chinese technical terms. As in the first edition, I have followed the principle of translating all Chinese terms except qi, yin and yang. Unlike the first edtion, however, I have come to believe that it is no longer necessary to capitalize most of these translated terms to show that they are being used in their traditional Chinese medical sense. The only exceptions are the names of the twelve organs of traditional Chinese medicine, where the possibility of confusion remains. By this I mean, e.g., that a condition of the Heart (upper case) in traditional medicine is not necessarily identical to heart (lower case) disease in modern biomedicine. Capitalization here should resolve any doubt about which heart is meant.

For those readers who are more familiar with the Chinese names for certain terms, I have provided in the back of this book a short glossary with *pinyin* transliteration and Chinese characters.

Foreword

From the scattered references to the tongue in the *Yellow Emperor's Inner Classic* to its fuller elaboration in the Ming and Qing dynasties, tongue diagnosis became an essential part of the traditional literate medicine of China. More recently, several important books have been published in the People's Republic of China that have drawn upon and systematized the material from the older periods.

This first appearance in English of a systematic presentation of Chinese tongue diagnosis is an important contribution to the transmission of medical knowledge from East to West. Giovanni Maciocia, one of Europe's most respected teachers and practitioners of Chinese medicine, has performed a valuable service for all of us in the West who practice, teach or are learning the traditional medicine of the Orient. Taking several important Chinese textbooks as a basis, he has crafted an entirely new work that is a clear, precise and accurate description of this important pillar of Chinese medical examination. This new book, which is of considerable theoretical interest, has also been informed with the clinical expertise of Giovanni's many prominent mentors. The book demonstrates a clinical sensitivity that is uniquely Giovanni Maciocia's and reflects his own extensive clinical work in both the West and China. The color plates and case histories are a welcome amplification of the text and an important guide for clinical practice. They are valuable not only for their crispness and precision but also because they are drawn from the types of patients that Western practitioners most often see.

Many scholars have noted that throughout history medical knowledge and resources have been transferred between cultures in mutual contact.[1] This process can be slow, as between India and China,[2] or rapid, as the introduction of Western medicine into the largest cities of China in the nineteenth century. In either case, it always involves elements of confusion and chaos which can lead to unsuccessful grafts, such as acupuncture in 19th century Europe[3] or Greek medicine in Tang dynasty China.[4] Giovanni Maciocia's lucid presentation of Chinese tongue diagnosis in this book will undoubtedly help to make the process of adapting China's medical legacy to Western needs much easier, orderly and more enduring.

Ted Kaptchuk
Boston

NOTES

1. Paul U. Unschuld, "Western Medicine and Traditional Healing Systems: Competition, Cooperation or Integration?" *Ethics, Science and Medicine* 3, no. 1 (May 1976): 1-20.
2. Paul U. Unschuld, "The Chinese Reception of Indian Medicine in the First Millennium A.D." *Bulletin of the History of Medicine* 53, no. 3 (Fall 1979): 329-45.
3. John S. Haller, "Acupuncture in Nineteenth Century Western Medicine." *New York State Journal of Medicine* 73 (May 1973): 1213-21.
4. Edward H. Schafer, *The Golden Peaches of Samarkand: A Study of T'ang Exotics.* (Berkeley: University of California Press, 1963).

Acknowledgments

This book would not have been possible without the assistance of many teachers, colleagues and friends.

Dr. Su Xin-Ming of the Nanjing College of Traditional Chinese Medicine taught me the art of Chinese diagnosis during my two stays in China. I am indebted to him for communicating his knowledge and skills to me with infinite patience and fatherly affection.

To Dr. J.H.F. Shen I owe a great deal, particularly in regard to tongue diagnosis. During his seminars in London and private communications in Boston, he generously taught me many of the fundamental aspects of tongue diagnosis as well as some more unusual ways of looking at the tongue which were peculiar to his rich experience.

Ted Kaptchuk provided my first exposure to traditional Chinese medicine and the fundamentals of tongue diagnosis. His comments and support throughout the compilation of the manuscript were a source of great encouragement and inspiration.

Dr. Chen Jing-Hua, vice-director of the Friendship Hospital in Beijing, taught me diagnosis of the underside of the tongue by examining the veins. I am grateful to her for sharing this information with me.

I am indebted to Michael McIntyre for reading the proofs and for his expert advice, and to Hugh O'Connor, John O'Connor and Dan Bensky of Eastland Press for their capable editing. Linda Upton prepared the illustrations for which I am grateful.

I would also like to acknowledge the work of the authors of the modern Chinese texts noted in the bibliography, especially *Tongue Diagnosis in Chinese Medicine,* from which I drew much inspiration and knowledge.

Finally, I am deeply indebted to my wife Christine for her constant support and encouragement without which this book would not have been realized.

1
History of
Chinese Tongue Diagnosis

From its inception, Chinese medicine has paid close attention to the external appearance and demeanor of the patient. It has always regarded the external appearance as a reflection of internal processes. From oracle bone inscriptions we know that at least one aspect of this approach, diagnosis by inspection of the tongue, was important as far back as the Shang dynasty (c. 16th CENTURY B.C.–1066 B.C.).[1]

WARRING STATES PERIOD (403 B.C–221 B.C.)

Although politically chaotic, the Warring States period was a time of great economic and cultural development. It was during this era that all the major schools of Chinese philosophical thought (including Taoism, Confucianism and Naturalism[2]) arose, each of which has deeply influenced Chinese society and politics to the present day. Fundamental theories of Chinese medicine, notably the concepts of yin-yang and the five phases, were also developed in this period. Important medical texts include the *Yellow Emperor's Inner Classic*,[3] the *Classic of Difficulties*,[4] and the *Divine Husbandman's Classic of the Materia Medica*.

Tongue diagnosis was an integral part of Chinese medical practice at this time. Several passages from the *Yellow Emperor's Inner Classic* mention specific tongue conditions and their significance in the clinic:

> If the tongue is loose, there is drooling and the patient is irritable, choose the leg lesser yin [Kidney channel].[5]

> When the Heart pulse is hard and long, then the tongue curls up and the patient cannot speak.[6]

> If the qi of the leg terminal yin [Liver] is exhausted . . . the lips turn blue and the tongue curls.[7]

These excerpts reveal that diagnosis was based primarily on the shape of the tongue and that the tongue's appearance was correlated with the pulse and facial diagnosis. The *Yellow Emperor's Inner Classic* also mentions several other types of tongue body shapes including rolled, stiff, withered and short. These descriptive types are still in use today.

Although the shape of the tongue is the focus of discussion, there are also a few references to the color of the tongue's coating:

> When the Lungs are invaded by heat...tiny hairs stand up, the patient has an aversion to cold, the tongue coating is yellow and the body hot[8].

> When the yang qi is abundant and the yin qi is insufficient, the insufficient yin qi leads to internal heat and the abundant yang qi leads to external heat... The tongue will be burnt, the lips withered and the skin as dry as dried meat.[9]

These passages show that a connection had already been recognized between heat and a yellow tongue coating.

Other passages in the *Yellow Emperor's Inner Classic* indicate that observation of the tongue can also be used to judge the prognosis of the patient's condition. For example, "If hemiplegia occurs on the left side in men and on the right side in women...[and] if the patient can still talk and move the tongue, he or she will recover within one month."[10] In other words, the prognosis is good if the tongue can move and poor if the tongue is stiff.

Thus the *Yellow Emperor's Inner Classic* contains the first important elements of tongue diagnosis — particularly in its analysis of the shape of the tongue — but no systematic description of the body of the tongue or the color of its coating.

HAN DYNASTY (206 B.C.–220 A.D.)

This era witnessed the synthesis of many of the diverse strands of Chinese medical theory. The most important contributions to tongue diagnosis were made by Zhang Zhong-Jing, author of the *Discussion of Cold-induced Disorders* and the *Essentials of the Golden Cabinet*. Zhang correlated alterations in tongue body and coating color with pathological changes:

> A yellow tongue coating and a feeling of fullness in the intestines indicates excess heat. If purging is applied and the heat is cleared, the yellow coating disappears.[11]

> In yang brightness disorders with constipation, abdominal fullness and vomiting the tongue has a white coating.[12]

> In the absence of heat signs . . . the patient is quiet and the tongue has a slippery coating. . .[13]

Not only did Zhang analyze changes in tongue coating, but also those in tongue body color. For example, "If the patient has fullness of the chest, dry lips and the tongue body color is bluish. . .it indicates stasis of blood."[14]

Zhang was also the first to observe the relationship between the thickness of the tongue coating and the strength of the pathogenic factors, as well as the relationship of white or yellow coating to cold or hot conditions.

Zhang's analysis of tongue coating provides an important basis for differentiating disease patterns. The *Discussion of Cold-induced Disorders* became the undisputed authoritative text for the differentiation and treatment of diseases caused by externally-contracted cold. Historically, Zhang lived in an era characterized by the prevalence of such diseases, in contrast to later epochs characterized by diseases from externally-contracted heat such as smallpox, measles and scarlet fever.[15]

SUI AND TANG DYNASTIES (581–907)

During the Sui and Tang dynasties there was unprecedented economic and cultural development in Chinese society. This was the period in which Buddhism reached its height of popularity in China. In the field of medicine, too, important developments occurred. The Imperial Medical College was first established, fostering the clinical application of acupuncture and herbal medicine.

With respect to tongue diagnosis, the most important documents of this period are the *Discussion of the Origins and Symptoms of Diseases*[16] by Chao Yuan-Fang, which was printed in the early seventh century, and the *Thousand Ducat Prescriptions*[17] by Sun Si-Miao (581-682), printed in 652. These works further elaborate upon the application of tongue body shape, color and coating in the differentiation of disease patterns. Chao referred to the appearance of the tongue in many passages of his book, a few examples of which follow:

> In Kidney yin deficiency the mouth is hot, the tongue dry and the patient thirsty.[18]

> For those with diseases from heat in the Lungs . . . the top of the tongue will be yellow, the body hot . . . those whose tongues are 'burnt' black will die.[19]

> When there is no coating on top of the tongue, attacking methods [of treatment] cannot be used.[20]

Sun Si-Miao is by far the most famous physician of the early Tang period and his book had a tremendous influence on later generations of practitioners. He too made many observations about the tongue in his writings:

> If the tongue is stiff and the patient is unable to talk, the disease is in the Organs.[21]

> In extreme deficiency of the sinews . . . the tongue will be rolled.[22]

> In excess patterns of the Heart the tongue will be cracked.[23]

> If the yin Organs are hot the tongue will be ulcerated . . . if the yang Organs are cold the tongue will be contracted.[24]

If the tongue is rolled and contracted. . . [externally-contracted] pathogenic heat has injured the Spleen.[25]

When the Stomach is expended. . . the tongue is swollen.[26]

When there is dysentery-like diarrhea and the tongue is yellow and desiccated but the patient is not thirsty, it indicates excess in the chest.[27]

In thirsty patients the throat will be 'burnt' and this will result in a dry tongue.[28]

Both Chao and Sun paid particular attention to the appearance of the tongue in pregnant women. An example from Chao's book is illustrative: "When the fetus is restless. . . and the mother presents with a red face and a blue tongue, the child will die and the mother will live; if the mother's face is blue and her tongue is red and she drools, she will die and the child will live."[29]

SONG AND JIN DYNASTIES (960–1234)

The Song dynasty was a period of consolidation of Confucian philosophy and ideology in every aspect of Chinese society. It was during the Song that many of the theories of Chinese medicine were integrated into a unified system by the Neo-Confucianists, eclectic thinkers whose philosophy encompassed Taoism, Buddhism, Naturalism, Legalism and Mohism. This eclecticism extended to medicine as well.

Tongue diagnosis attracted the attention of many physicians and gradually became a subject of specialized study. Medical writers continued to record their diagnostic observations:

If there is restlessness, a feeling of oppression in the chest, dry tongue, thirst and a deep, slippery pulse, it indicates a heat pattern.[30]

Dry mouth, dry tongue and a slow, deep pulse in both the front and rear positions indicates disease of the lesser yin [Kidney].[31]

Toward the end of the Jin dynasty, Li Dong-Yuan wrote an important book, *Discussion of the Spleen and Stomach*,[32] in which he advanced the idea that the Spleen and Stomach are the most important Organs of the body and that treatment should almost always be directed at these Organs. With respect to tongue diagnosis, he gave particular prominence to the dry tongue, which he related to various etiological factors. According to Li, a dry tongue with dry throat is due to an irregular diet and overwork; a dry tongue with chest and hypochondriac pain is caused by stagnation of Liver qi from emotional problems; and a dry tongue with a bitter taste in the mouth is symptomatic of Heart fire. These statements are interesting as examples of the diagnostic method of Chinese medicine by which one symptom (a dry tongue in this case) must be evaluated in the context of other symptoms and signs, with a different clinical significance attributed to different combinations of such symptoms.

It was also Li Dong-Yuan who made the correlation between a dry or wet tongue and excess/deficiency or yang/yin conditions (SEE CHAPTER 4).

YUAN DYNASTY (1279–1368)

During the Yuan dynasty tongue diagnosis became a separate specialty in medical studies. Many important books appeared which became the foundation for all subsequent literature on this subject.

A practitioner known only by his surname, Ao, wrote the *Record of the Golden Mirror*[33] toward the beginning of the Yuan dynasty. This is the first book devoted entirely to tongue diagnosis and is primarily concerned with its use in connection with cold-induced disorders, as described in Zhang Zhong-Jing's *Discussion of Cold-induced Disorders*. It contained twelve illustrations. This book, however, did not achieve wide circulation. Later in the Yuan dynasty, another physician named Du Qing-Bi read the book and appreciated its value. He edited it, added twenty-four new illustrations and published the revised work in 1341 under the title, *Ao's Record of the Golden Mirror of Cold -induced Disorders*.[34] The tongue body colors discussed are pale, red and blue. Alterations in the surface of the tongue include red prickles, red "stars," cracks and others. Coating colors are described as white, yellow, gray or black. Tongue shapes are differentiated as swollen, flabby, prickly, deviated and others. Each illustration is accompanied by an explanation as well as the pulse and pattern connected with that tongue condition. Each pattern is analyzed in terms of deficiency or excess and hot or cold influences. The cause of the disease, pathology and herbal treatment are indicated. In addition, Du Qing-Bi discussed the severity of the disease and prognosis from a clinical perspective. The book is thus a very thorough clinical manual with an emphasis on tongue diagnosis.

MING AND QING DYNASTIES (1368-1911)

During the Ming dynasty several books on tongue diagnosis were published, all modeled on *Ao's Record of the Golden Mirror of Cold-induced Disorders*. Among them, Shen Dou-Yuan's *Essential Methods of Observation of the Tongue in Cold-induced Disorders*[35] is the most prominent. In this book, 135 types of tongues are described.

During the Ming and (especially) the Qing dynasties, there was a high incidence of epidemics of exanthematous diseases such as smallpox, scarlet fever, chicken-pox and measles. These diseases are regarded in Chinese medicine as being caused by externally-contracted heat. The study of these diseases involved a difficult break with the tradition of the *Discussion of Cold-induced Disorders* of the Han dynasty. This book had become gospel for the differentiation and treatment of externally-contracted diseases, whether from cold or heat. Indeed, a common maxim held that "The method should not depart from that of the *Discussion of Cold-induced Disorders;* the prescription should follow that of [Zhang] Zhong-Jing."

The first dissent against such dogma was voiced as early as the Song dynasty when He Jian said that one could not use the prescriptions of the *Discussion of Cold-induced Disorders* for certain diseases caused by externally-contracted heat. Dr. He's dissent became so famous that a saying was coined: "In diseases from externally-contracted cold, follow [Zhang] Zhong-Jing; in diseases from externally-contracted heat, follow He Jian."[36] However it was not until the Qing dynasty, in response to the epidemics of that era, that a comprehensive and systematic theory of differentiation, diagnosis and treatment of disease from externally-contracted heat was developed. This was reflected in the field of tongue diagnosis by a very detailed study and analysis of red tongues. Historically, therefore, the differentiation of various types of red tongues was very much a product of the differentiation of diseases due to externally-contracted heat that was so prevalent during the Qing dynasty.

Several comprehensive works on tongue diagnosis were written during the Qing period. In the early years of this dynasty, Zhang Dan-Xian wrote the *Mirror of the Tongue in Cold-induced Disorders.*[37] This book contains 120 illustrations and is based on the *Essential Methods* from the Ming dynasty. However, toward the end of the Qing, Fu Song-Yuan wrote *A Collection of Tongues and Coatings,*[38] which departs from the tradition of discussing tongue diagnosis only in the light of cold-induced disorders. Included in this work are considerations of heat-induced and various other disorders. Fu also made an important departure from prior texts which usually classified tongues according to coating color. Instead, he classified tongues according to body color, regarding this as a more significant factor than the color of the tongue's coating. This view prevails today. In his book, Fu described eight primary tongue body colors: white, pale white, pale red, true red, deep red, purple, blue and black.

In 1906, Liang Te-Yan wrote the *Differentiation of Syndromes by Examination of the Tongue*[39] in which 148 types of tongues were described and illustrated.

Apart from these books which were devoted entirely to tongue diagnosis, other general books on Chinese medicine deserve mention here for their importance in this field.

The famous Ming physician Zhang Jie-Bing, also known as Zhang Jing-Yue, wrote the *Complete Treatises of [Zhang] Jing-Yue.*[40] One chapter, entitled "Tongue Color Differentiation," elaborated upon tongue body color in relation to the differentiation of disease patterns. Chen Shi-Duo wrote the *Secret Record of the Stone Room,*[41] one chapter of which is entitled "Experience Regarding Tongue Differentiation in Externally-contracted Diseases." In this chapter, Chen discussed how changes of the tongue coating reflect pathological changes in diseases from externally-contracted heat. He contended that regardless of whether the condition is mild or severe, deficient or excessive, or whether there is dampness or exhaustion of body fluids, it will always be identifiable by changes in the tongue coating.

Ye Tian-Shi, a very influential 18th-century physician, was the foremost authority on the study of diseases from externally-contracted heat. In 1746 he wrote the *Discussion of Warm-febrile Diseases.*[42] Ye introduced the principles of differentiation according to the four levels of disease, which became the foundation for the differentiation and treatment of warm-febrile diseases to this day (SEE APPENDIX II). He correlated the "true" or "false" coating (i.e., coating with or without "root") with conditions of deficiency or excess. He also analyzed tongue coating changes in warm-febrile diseases in great detail. Ye attached considerable importance to tongue diagnosis, commenting that "every clinical manifestation is reflected on the tongue."[43]

Wu Ju-Tong wrote the *Systematic Differentiation of Febrile Diseases*[44] in 1798. This is an elaboration of the work of Ye Tian-Shi, and introduced the principles of differentiation according to the three burners, which integrates Dr. Ye's four levels approach (SEE APPENDIX III). Wu also expanded the use of tongue diagnosis in cases of warm-febrile diseases.

The late-Qing physician Shi Shi-Nan, in a book entitled *Medical Sources,*[45] wrote a chapter entitled "Differentiation of Syndromes According to Tongue Coating in Various Diseases." In this chapter, Shi analyzed the physiological process of tongue coating formation and described how external pathogenic factors are reflected in pathological changes of the coating.

REPUBLIC OF CHINA (1911–1949)

During the Republican period traditional Chinese medicine probably reached its nadir. It was almost banned by the Nationalist government. By this time modern biomedicine was firmly established as the official medicine of China, even though biomedical facilities in the countryside were practically nonexistent. Traditional Chinese medicine came to be looked down upon by the Westernized educated classes. Consequently, very few new contributions to the development of traditional Chinese medicine were made.

PEOPLE'S REPUBLIC OF CHINA (1949–)

A vast improvement in the health of the Chinese people, and in the provision of health care, has taken place since the founding of the People's Republic. There has been a renaissance of traditional Chinese medicine, which is now studied in parallel with its Western counterpart. As a result, the study of Chinese medicine has made great strides. There are many colleges of traditional Chinese medicine with five- or six-year curricula, and many large hospitals devoted entirely to Chinese medicine. An enormous amount of research is being conducted to investigate the use of acupuncture and herbal medicine, and many books have been published since 1950 regarding both the modern and traditional aspects of Chinese medicine.

Many new books on tongue diagnosis have been published in recent years, most notably *Tongue Diagnosis in Chinese Medicine*. This work is a systematic discussion of all aspects of tongue diagnosis and draws upon all the previous classics. Another important textbook, *Chinese Medical Diagnosis*, contains an excellent chapter on tongue diagnosis. In particular, it provides a fine discussion of the clinical significance of coating, with or without "root." It contains twelve color photographs.

Chinese medical journals regularly carry articles on tongue diagnosis, often discussing the integration of Western and Chinese diagnostic techniques. For example, one article[46] demonstrated that a traditional Chinese disorder may occur across many different Western-defined diseases. In this study of 108 cases with bluish purple tongue, each case was found to involve stasis of Liver blood, irrespective of the diagnosis given the patient by modern biomedicine. Another article[47] stated that all 39 cases of chronic infectious hepatitis in the study were characterized by a yellow, greasy tongue coating reflecting damp-heat in the Liver and Gallbladder. This shows that there can be a congruence between Chinese and modern biomedicine.

Due to the close integration of traditional Chinese and modern biomedicine in China, many studies have been carried out showing how the appearance of the tongue is closely correlated with various patterns of biomedically-defined diseases. Thus, tongue diagnosis can give pointers of treatment not only in traditional Chinese medicine, but also modern biomedicine. For example, an article[48] in the *Journal of Chinese Medicine* reported on the observation of 524 patients suffering from chronic hepatitis B. Results showed, on the basis of tongue appearance, that 32% presented with damp-heat, 22% with stagnation of qi and accumulation of dampness, 22% with Liver-yin deficiency, 14% with stasis of blood, 7% with deficiency of qi and accumulation of dampness, and 3% with Spleen and Kidney yang deficiency.

Another article[49] reported that changes of the tongue body in diabetic patients are in relation with blood viscosity: a dark-red tongue indicates an increase in blood viscosity.

Research in China also shows that the appearance of the tongue can be correlated with biomedically-defined diseases rather than Chinese disease-symptoms, e.g., "atrophic gastritis" rather than "epigastric pain". An article[50] in the *Journal of Chinese Medicine* reported that, in the context of gastric signs and symptoms, a yellow-thick coating may indicate gastritis; a partially peeled coating may indicate chronic atrophic gastritis; brown spots may denote atrophic gastritis; and a green coating with purple spots on the tongue body may indicate carcinoma of the stomach.

Tongue diagnosis is, of course, taught at all colleges of traditional Chinese medicine in China. Visual aids such as slides or wax models of all types of tongues are often used.

It is difficult to predict how tongue diagnosis will continue to evolve in modern China. The country's recent history has witnessed many radical swings in political line, all of which have had repercussions in the official support given to traditional Chinese medicine and the delivery of medical care. For example, during the Cultural Revolution (1966-1976) most of the traditional theories of Chinese medicine were rejected as being remnants of "feudal thinking" at worst, or of "primitive naive materialism" at best. The situation has changed dramatically since then, and continues to change very rapidly from year to year. There is now a renewed appreciation for study of the classics and the traditional theories of Chinese medicine. An example in point is the enormous interest and research in *qi gong*, the ancient Taoist breathing exercises used to promote health.

The need to train vast numbers of doctors and medical workers in China has often led to the simplification of traditional medicine, sometimes to the detriment of its more subtle theoretical aspects. With respect to tongue diagnosis, this has meant that the diagnostic standard of newly-trained doctors tends to be very basic, while the finer points of diagnosis are only practiced by the older doctors. My own view is that the teaching institutions of Chinese medicine must harmonize the need for didactic simplification and standardization with the need for research on more subtle and traditional aspects in this field. If this balance can be successfully achieved, tongue diagnosis will continue to advance as a vital aspect of Chinese medical theory and practice.

NOTES

1. Chen Ze-Lin, "Overview of the History of Tongue Diagnosis." *Chinese Journal of Medical History (Zhong hua yi shi za zhi)* 12 (1982): 1-3.

2. I call "naturalism" the philosophy of the "Yin Yang School" which flourished during the Warring States period. The main exponent of this school was Zou Yan (c. 350 B.C.-270 B.C.). This is the school that elaborated the theories of yin-yang and the five phases, which became the theoretical foundations of Chinese medicine. For an excellent discussion of the theories of this school, see Joseph Needham's *Science and Civilization in China* II (Cambridge: Cambridge University Press, 1956), pp. 232-65.

3. The *Yellow Emperor's Inner Classic (Huang di nei jing)* is the earliest classic of Chinese medicine, most of which was written during the Warring States period. It is traditionally attributed to the mythical Yellow Emperor (who supposedly reigned about 2700 B.C.) but it was obviously written no earlier than 300 B.C. by several different authors, and was subsequently edited several times. The edition available today was compiled by Wang Bing in 762 A.D. The *Yellow Emperor's Inner Classic* consists of two parts, *Simple Questions (Su wen)* and *Spiritual Axis (Ling shu)*, each of which contains eighty-one chapters. *Simple Questions* deals with the theory of Chinese medicine including physiology, pathology, causes of disease, channel pathways and diagnosis. *Spiritual Axis* is devoted to acupuncture and moxibustion and describes the nine types of needles, needle technique, functions of the points and the treatment of several diseases.

4. The *Classic of Difficulties (Nan jing)* was also written during the Warring States period, or perhaps during the Han dynasty. Formerly believed to be the work of the famous physician Bian Que (6th century B.C.), it is now thought by many to have been written by Qin Yue-Ren in the 3rd century B.C. The latter used the pseudonym Bian Que to gain respectability for his work. This was a common custom in ancient China. (For more information, see Joseph Needham and Lu Gwei-Djen, *Celestial Lancets* [Cambridge: Cambridge University Press, 1980], pp. 79-88 and pp. 114-15.) *Classic of Difficulties* consists of eighty-one chapters and elucidates certain subjects that were only briefly described in the *Yellow Emperor's Inner Classic*. It is regarded as an important text for several reasons. It established the practice of taking the pulse at the radial artery,

dealt with the concept of the gate of vitality and introduced rules on the use of the five command or transporting points *(shu xue)* of each channel. It also introduced the concept of tonification and sedation points according to the generating cycle of the five phases.

5. *Classic of the Spiritual Axis (Ling shu jing)* (Beijing: People's Medical Publishing House, 1963), chap. 21, p. 56.

6. *Yellow Emperor's Inner Classic: Simple Questions (Huang di nei jing su wen)* (Beijing: People's Medical Publishing House, 1963), chap. 17, p. 98.

7. *Classic of the Spiritual Axis,* chap. 10, p. 30.

8. *Yellow Emperor's Inner Classic: Simple Questions,* chap. 32, p. 186.

9. *Classic of the Spiritual Axis,* chap. 75, p. 134.

10. *Yellow Emperor's Inner Classic: Simple Questions,* chap. 48, p. 264.

11. He Ren, ed., *Essentials of the Golden Cabinet: A New Explanation (Jin gui yao lue xin jie)* (Zhejiang: Zhejiang Scientific Publishing House, 1981), chap. 10, p. 65.

12. Cold-induced Diseases Research and Teaching Group of the Nanjing College of Traditional Chinese Medicine, ed., *Discussion of Cold-induced Disorders with Explanations (Shang han lun yi shi)* (Shanghai: Shanghai Scientific Publishing House, 1980), p. 948.

13. *Discussion of Cold-induced Disorders,* p. 703.

14. *Essentials of the Golden Cabinet,* chap. 16, p. 138.

15. There is evidence that diseases characterized by rash and fever did not exist in China during the Han dynasty. They appeared later and their incidence increased until reaching a peak during the Qing dynasty. This was due to several factors including increased population density and urbanization (important factors in the spreading of epidemics); increased trade within China and with foreign peoples (contact with new diseases); the shifting of the center of Chinese civilization from the cold Yellow River basin of the north to the hot Yangzi River valley of the south (change in climate); and the Mongol invasion of the 13th century (spreading of the plague). These factors led to an increase in epidemics of diseases from externally-contracted heat after the Han dynasty, particularly during the late Ming and early Qing dynasties (see also Appendix II). A fascinating account of the influence of epidemics on the social and political history of mankind is the book by W. H. McNeil, *Plagues and Peoples* (New York: Penguin Books, 1976).

16. Chao Yuan-Fang, *Discussion of the Origins and Symptoms of Diseases (Zhu bing yuan hou lun).*

17. Sun Si-Miao, *Thousand Ducat Prescriptions (Qian jin yao fang).*

18. *Discussion of the Origins and Symptoms of Diseases,* sec. 41. Cited in Beijing College of Traditional Chinese Medicine, *Tongue Diagnosis in Chinese Medicine (Zhong yi she zhen)* (Beijing: People's Medical Publishing House, 1976), p. 3.

19. *Discussion of the Origins and Symptoms of Diseases,* sec. 8. Cited in *Tongue Diagnosis in Chinese Medicine,* p 2.

20. *Discussion of the Origins and Symptoms of Diseases,* sec. 7. Cited in *Tongue Diagnosis in Chinese Medicine,* p 3.

21. *Thousand Ducat Prescriptions,* sec. 8. Cited in *Tongue Diagnosis in Chinese Medicine,* p. 3.

22. *Thousand Ducat Prescriptions*, sec. 11, chap. 4. Cited in *Tongue Diagnosis in Chinese Medicine*, p 3.

23. *Thousand Ducat Prescriptions*, sec. 13, chap. 1. Cited in *Tongue Diagnosis in Chinese Medicine*, p 3.

24. *Thousand Ducat Prescriptions*, sec. 14, chap. 3. Cited in *Tongue Diagnosis in Chinese Medicine*, p 3.

25. *Thousand Ducat Prescriptions*, sec. 15, chap. 1. Cited in *Tongue Diagnosis in Chinese Medicine*, p 3.

26. *Thousand Ducat Prescriptions*, sec. 16, chap. 1. Cited in *Tongue Diagnosis in Chinese Medicine*, p 3.

27. *Thousand Ducat Prescriptions*, sec. 15. Cited in *Tongue Diagnosis in Chinese Medicine*, p. 3.

28. *Thousand Ducat Prescriptions*, sec. 26. Cited in *Tongue Diagnosis in Chinese Medicine*, p. 3.

29. *Discussion of the Origins and Symptoms of Diseases*, sec. 41. Cited in *Tongue Diagnosis in Chinese Medicine*, p. 3. A similar passage from *Thousand Ducat Prescriptions*, sec. 2, chap. 6, is also cited on p. 3 of the same source.

30. Guo Yong, *Discussion of Cold-induced Disorders with Lost Passages Replaced (Shang han bu wang lun)* (date unknown). Cited in *Tongue Diagnosis in Chinese Medicine*, p. 4.

31. *Discussion of Cold-induced Disorders with Lost Passages Replaced*. Cited in *Tongue Diagnosis in Chinese Medicine*, p. 4.

32. Li Dong-Yuan, *Discussion of the Spleen and Stomach (Pi wei lun)* (1249).

33. Ao, *Record of the Golden Mirror (Jin jing lu)* (c. 1280).

34. Du Qing-Bi, *Ao's Record of the Golden Mirror of Cold-induced Disorders (Ao shi shang han jin jing lu)* (1341).

35. Shen Dou-Yuan, *Essential Methods of Observation of the Tongue in Cold-induced Disorders (Shang han guan xin fa)* (date unknown).

36. Nanjing College of Traditional Chinese Medicine, *Study of Febrile Diseases (Wen bing xue)* (Shanghai: Shanghai Scientific Publishing House, 1978), p. 12.

37. Zhang Dan-Xian, *Mirror of the Tongue in Cold-induced Disorders (Shang han she jian)* (1668).

38. Fu Song-Yuan, *A Collection of Tongues and Coatings (She tai tong zhi)* (1874).

39. Liang Te-Yan, *Differentiation of Syndromes by Examination of the Tongue (She jian bian zheng)* (1906).

40. Zhang Jie-Bing, *The Complete Treatises of [Zhang] Jing-Yue (Jing-yue quan shu)* (1634).

41. Chen Shi-Duo, *Secret Record of the Stone Room (She shi mi lu)* (1687).

42. Ye Tian-Shi, *Discussion of Warm-febrile Diseases (Wen re lun)* (1746).

43. Chen Zi-Lin, "Overview of the History of Tongue Diagnosis." *Chinese Journal of Medical History (Zhong hua yi shi za zhi)* 12 (1982): 1-4.

44. Wu Ju-Tong, *Systematic Differentiation of Febrile Diseases (Wen bing tiao bian)* (1798).

45. Shi Shi-Nan, *Medical Sources (Yi yuan)* (1891).

46. Hu Qing-Fu and Chen Ze-Lin, "Analysis and Discussion of the Clinical Materials Relating to 108 Cases of Bluish Purple Tongues." *Journal of Traditional Chinese Medicine (Zhong yi za zhi)* 24, no. 6 (1983): 67.

47. Wang Cheng-Bai, "Differentiation of Syndromes and Discussion of Treatment for Yellow, Greasy Tongue Coatings Accompanying Chronic Hepatitis." *Journal of Traditional Chinese Medicine (Zhong yi za zhi)* 25, no. 4 (1984): 26.

48. Chen Han-Cheng, "Tongue Diagnosis and Identification of Patterns in Chronic Hepatitis B." *Journal of Traditional Chinese Medicine (Zhong yi za zhi)* 29, no. 4 (1988): 53.

49. Zhao Rong-Lai et al, "Computer Scanning and Classification of Tongue Body and Coating." *Journal of Traditional Chinese Medicine (Zhong yi za zhi)* 30, no.2 (1989): 47.

50. Dai Hao-Liang, "A Comparative Study between the Tongue Appearance and Fibre-optic Gastroscopy." *Journal of Traditional Chinese Medicine (Zhong yi za zhi)* 25, no.10 (1984): 74.

2

Tongue Examination: An Overview

WESTERN ANATOMY OF THE TONGUE[1]

The tongue is composed of skeletal muscle covered with mucous membrane. Several muscles that originate in the bones of the skull insert into the tongue. The elevations on the tongue's surface are called papillae, which are folds of the cellular top layer of the tongue (ILLUSTRATION 2-1). There are five types of papillae:

- Foliate
- Filiform
- Fungiform
- Vallate
- Circumvallate

The tip and dorsum of the tongue are covered by a mass of filiform papillae interspersed with fungiform papillae. At the very back, on the root of the tongue, there is a set of V-shaped large circumvallate papillae which have a protective function in preventing the swallowing of bitter-poisonous substances. These large papillae, which are visible only if the patient protrudes the tongue to its utmost, are an anatomical feature of the normal tongue and should not be mistakenly interpreted as "red spots." As we will see later, Chinese tongue diagnosis mostly puts the emphasis on two types of papillae: the filiform papillae forming the "coating" and the fungiform papillae that form the actual surface of the tongue body and become "red points or spots" in pathological conditions.

Between 16 and 96 years of age the epithelial layer of cells on the surface of the tongue undergoes a 30% reduction in thickness, whilst the basal cell layer remains the same. This is interesting as it coincides with the progressive reduction in tongue coating associated with old age; this is due to a high prevalence

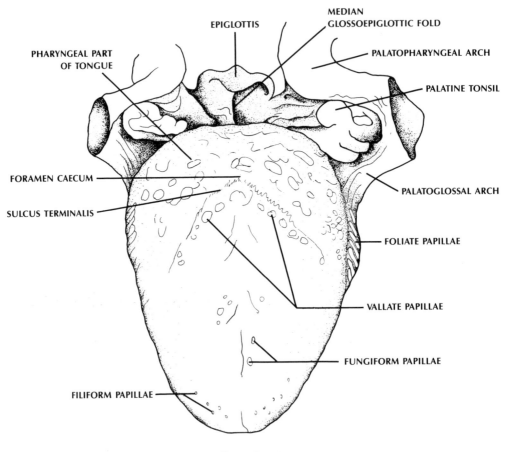

PHARYNGEAL PART
OF TONGUE

EPIGLOTTIS

MEDIAN
GLOSSOEPIGLOTTIC FOLD

PALATOPHARYNGEAL ARCH

PALATINE TONSIL

FORAMEN CAECUM

SULCUS TERMINALIS

PALATOGLOSSAL ARCH

FOLIATE PAPILLAE

VALLATE PAPILLAE

FUNGIFORM PAPILLAE

FILIFORM PAPILLAE

Illustration 2-1

of yin deficiency which has been recognized in Chinese medicine.

Considering the embryological development of the tongue, in the very early embryo the head part of the embryonic area folds over to enclose the primitive foregut between the amniotic cavity and the primitive pericardium (ILLUSTRATION 2-2). The tongue develops in the area of mandibular growth between the primitive mouth and the thorax. The developing tongue separates the primitive mouth opening from the pericardium and primitive cardiac development (ILLUSTRATION 2-3). This is very interesting as it seems to coincide with the correlation in Chinese medicine between the tongue and the Heart/Pericardium.

The tongue doubles in length, width and thickness between birth and adolescence, and its size is proportional to the size of the head under normal conditions.

TONGUE DIAGNOSIS: STRENGTHS AND WEAKNESSES

Tongue diagnosis has several distinctions which make it of critical importance in Chinese diagnostics. In some respects it is more reliable than pulse diagnosis.

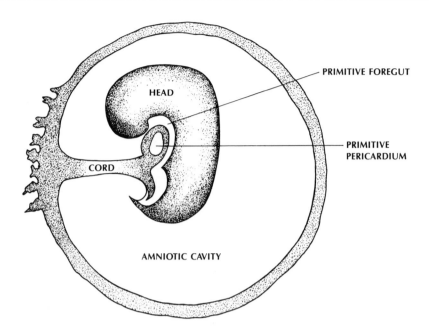

PRIMITIVE FOREGUT

HEAD

PRIMITIVE PERICARDIUM

CORD

AMNIOTIC CAVITY

Illustration 2-2

It is therefore useful at this point to review both its strengths and deficiencies. First, the tongue body color almost always reflects the true condition of the patient, especially in terms of the eight principles identification of patterns. The complex of symptoms and signs in a patient's presentation may often be contradictory. For example, a patient may display some symptoms of interior cold, such as a pale tongue body, loose stool and chills, and yet have a rapid pulse, which is a sign of heat. In such situations the color of the tongue body is the most reliable sign and will always point to the true condition. One reason for this is that the tongue body and coating colors are relatively unaffected by short-term events or recent changes. For instance, a patient may have had a disturbing experience just before the consultation; this would probably make the pulse faster and slightly tight, but it would not change the tongue body or coating color. (Of course, persisting emotional problems will definitely affect the tongue's appearance, particularly the tongue body color.) Similarly, a patient who has just taken vigorous exercise will have a rapid pulse, but the tongue color will be relatively unaffected.

Second, the tongue's appearance is a most useful gauge for monitoring the improvement or decline of the patient's condition. For this purpose, the tongue body color is more useful in chronic conditions, while the tongue coating is generally more useful in acute conditions.

Third, the topography of the tongue, i.e., the correspondence of different areas of the tongue to different Organs, is a subject of fairly general agreement.

Fourth, tongue diagnosis is relatively objective in comparison with other techniques. While there may be disagreement about whether a certain pulse is "tight" or "wiry," if a tongue is dark red, there can be little doubt that it is so. However

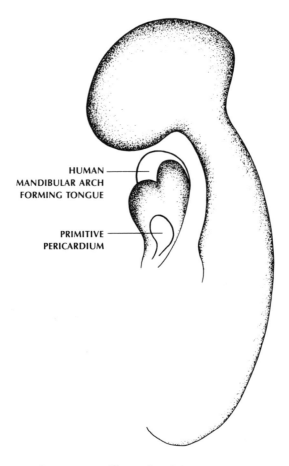

HUMAN
MANDIBULAR ARCH
FORMING TONGUE

PRIMITIVE
PERICARDIUM

Illustration 2-3

it is important to remember that some shades of tongue body color can be rather subtle. For instance, the detection of the pale blue tongue body color requires some experience.

Finally, tongue diagnosis is rather easy to learn, at least compared to pulse diagnosis. Knowledge of this technique can be acquired by observing tongues in clinical practice, as well as by viewing visual aids such as video tapes and photographs.

The principal limitation of tongue diagnosis when compared with pulse diagnosis is its relative lack of precision. A practitioner of Chinese medicine experienced in the interpretation of the pulse can extract a lot of detailed information about a patient's condition, often identifying the source of a medical problem. However, a thick, sticky, yellow tongue coating with red spots on the root, while indicating the retention of damp-heat in the lower burner, does not by itself indicate whether the problem is in the Bladder, Intestines, Kidneys or Womb. This distinction can only be made if the pulse and other signs and symptoms are taken into account.

A more detailed exposition of the significance and use of tongue diagnosis in clinical practice can be found in chapter 8, where there is a specific discussion of the use of tongue diagnosis in complex and contradictory situations.

EXAMINING THE TONGUE

There are several important points to remember when examining the tongue in order to avoid false or distorted findings.

Proper lighting is critical to a reliable examination. The best possible light is natural sunlight. Artificial light will never be entirely adequate. For this reason it is essential to examine the tongue as close to a window as possible. If tongue diagnosis must be conducted in artificial light, incandescent is preferable to fluorescent light, and a strong light is better than a weak one. If fluorescent lighting is used, it must be full-spectrum light. A tungsten halogen lamp is also ideal.

One should ask the patient to extend the tongue as much as possible, but without excessive force. This is important because using too much force to extend the tongue will change its shape and make it redder.

The patient should be asked to extend the tongue for a short time only, no more than 15-20 seconds. Prolonged extension of the tongue will tend to redden it, more quickly so on its tip. If a longer examination is required, one can ask the patient to withdraw the tongue, close the mouth and then extend it again. This can be done several times without affecting the tongue color.

It is also always necessary to take great care when evaluating the tongue body color. Although this is usually quite straightforward, it may be rather difficult in those cases when the shade of color is subtle. This is especially true of purple shades like pale purple, bluish purple and reddish purple. A blue tongue will in most cases not appear bright blue (although in a few cases it will), but rather a subtle, bluish shade.

The consumption of highly colored foods and sweets will affect tongue color. One should ensure that the patient has not consumed foods of this kind just prior to the examination.

Spicy foods such as pickles, cayenne pepper, and curry will tend to redden the tongue for a short time after consumption. Smoking tobacco tends to turn the coating of the tongue yellow.

Effect of Medicines on the Tongue

Medicines can also affect the appearance of the tongue. Medicinal drugs obviously have an effect on the tongue's appearance and it is important to be aware of these so as to avoid drawing wrong conclusions in your diagnosis.

Antibiotics

These affect the tongue very quickly. They generally cause the tongue to become peeled in patches, i.e., the coating falls off in small areas. This is a clear reflection of the fact that antibiotics tend to injure Stomach yin.

Not all antibiotics, however, affect the tongue to the same degree. Tetracyclines affect the tongue more than any other type of antibiotic. To a lesser extent, chloramphenicol, gentamicins and related aminoglycosides also cause the same tongue appearance. The effects on the tongue appear after 2-3 days of administration and persist for about two weeks after medication has stopped.

Corticosteroids

Oral steroids cause the tongue to become red and swollen after about one month of administration. Inhaled steroids have the same effect only after a much longer time of continued daily use.

Bronchodilators

Beta$_2$-adrenoceptor stimulants (salbutamol, terbutaline, etc.) may cause the tongue tip to become red after prolonged and continued use. Other bronchodilators such as Theophylline have an even stronger tendency to produce this effect after a shorter time.

Diuretics

Diuretics remove body fluids drastically and may therefore cause yin deficiency; however, this usually occurs only after prolonged use over some years. Their effect on the tongue over the long run is to make it peeled, reflecting the yin deficiency.

Anti-Inflammatory Agents

The two anti-inflammatory drugs which affect the tongue most are phenylbutazone and oxyphenbutazone. Even though these are anti-inflammatory agents, they paradoxically cause the appearance of red points and make the tongue body thinner. After prolonged use over some years, the tongue may become peeled.

Other anti-inflammatory agents which have similar effects, but to a lesser degree, include commonly-used nonsteroidal anti-inflammatory drugs such as ibuprofen, naproxen, ketoprofen, fenoprofen, azapropazone, and indomethacin.

Antineoplastics

Most cytotoxic drugs used in treating malignant disease cause the tongue to develop a very thick brown or even black and dry coating.

ASPECTS OF TONGUE DIAGNOSIS

To examine the tongue systematically, one must have a clear idea of what to look for. There are five primary aspects to observe, listed here in order of examination. Each is discussed at greater length in chapters 5 through 7 below.

Vitality of Color, or Tongue Spirit

The appearance of vitality indicates an essentially healthy condition. This quality is sometimes described as the "spirit" of the tongue to denote an apparent liveliness, irrespective of any coincident pathological signs. If the tongue has a vital color, the prognosis is good; if it has a dark and withered appearance, the prognosis is poor. A tongue with a vital color is sometimes described as a "tongue of life," and a tongue with a dark and withered appearance as a "tongue of death." The terms life and death in this context should not be taken literally; they simply denote the relative seriousness of the disease.

Of particular importance in analyzing the vitality of the color is the careful scrutiny of the root of the tongue. If the root has a good, vibrant color the prognosis is good no matter what the disease. If the root has a dark, dry and withered look, the prognosis is poor.

Body Color

Body color refers to the color of the tongue itself, beneath any coating. If the coating is extremely thick and covers the entire surface of the tongue, one should examine the color of the underside of the tongue to properly judge the body color.

The clinical significance of the tongue body color is that it reflects the condition of the yin Organs, blood and nutritive qi. Body color is the single most important aspect of observation. It almost always reflects the true condition of the body, irrespective of temporary conditions such as those resulting from recent physical exertion or emotional upset. For example, if the tongue body color is very dark red, the condition is certain to be one of intense heat in one or more Organs regardless of what other symptoms and signs may be present. If the tongue is very pale or nearly white, the condition is definitely one of severe yang or blood deficiency. Very often the other clinical signs and symptoms will be contradictory; in such cases, the tongue body color is the definitive indicator for the diagnosis. In terms of eight principles identification of patterns, it reflects hot and cold influences; deficiency of yin, yang, qi or blood; and stagnation.

Body Shape

Examination of the body shape must include consideration of the shape itself, the features of the tongue surface, the texture of the tongue body and any involuntary movements of the tongue.

Examining the shape involves observing whether the tongue is thin or swollen, long or short, and whether specific parts of the tongue are swollen.

Examining the features of the tongue surface means looking for such aberrations as cracks and ulcers.

Examining the texture means observing the extent to which the tongue body is supple or stiff.

Examining the movement of the tongue body involves watching for any movement of the tongue when it is extended. Movements may include quivering, trembling, side-to-side motion, curling in any direction or shifting to one side.

The clinical significance of the tongue shape is that it reflects the state of the Organs, qi and blood. It is particularly useful in differentiating conditions of excess and deficiency.

Tongue Coating

The coating should be observed systematically from the tip to the root in each of four aspects.

Coating color reflects the hot or cold influences more directly than any other aspect of tongue diagnosis. A white coating corresponds to cold and a yellow coating to heat.

Coating thickness reflects the strength of the pathogenic factors present in the body; the stronger the pathogenic factors, the thicker the coating. In terms of differentiation, it reflects conditions of excess or deficiency.

Coating distribution reflects the progression and location of the pathogenic factor in externally-contracted diseases. For internally-generated diseases it reflects the location of the pathogenic factor in accordance with the tongue topography outlined in chapter 4. In terms of differentiation, it reflects the interior or exterior location of the disease.

A tongue coating may be with or without "root." A coating with root (also called "true coating") is firmly implanted in the tongue surface and grows out of it just like grass grows from the soil. Such coating cannot be scraped off. A coating without root looks as if it is sprinkled upon the tongue surface instead of growing from it. It can be scraped off. The rooting of the coating directly reflects the strength of the body's qi. From the perspective of differentiation, it is a reliable indicator of excess or deficiency of qi.

Tongue Moisture

Examination of tongue moisture provides an indication of the status of the body's fluids. The normal tongue is only slightly moist. A dry tongue indicates insufficiency of body fluids, while a wet tongue indicates their accumulation. In terms of differentiation, tongue moisture reflects the relative state of yin/yang and hot/cold.

THE NORMAL TONGUE

The characteristics of the normal tongue are as follows:

1. *Spirit.* The normal tongue should have spirit; its color should be vibrant and vital, particularly on the root.

2. *Body color.* The color should be pale red and "fresh-looking," very much like a fresh piece of meat. The tongue is regarded in Chinese medicine as the off-shoot of the Heart, meaning that the condition of the Heart qi and blood is reflected there. A normal, fresh, pale red color of the tongue body indicates that the tongue is receiving an abundant supply of Heart blood. Among the yang Organs, the

Stomach is the one which most influences the tongue. The Stomach is responsible for the production of a normal tongue coating and also sends fluids up to the tongue, the color of which then tends to be paler than if the fluids are not reaching the tongue. The proper tongue color is therefore pale red, resulting from a normal supply of Heart blood and Stomach fluids.

3. *Body shape.* The normal tongue body is supple, neither too flabby nor too stiff. It is not cracked, does not tremble or quiver when extended, and is neither swollen nor thin. It has no ulcers.

4. *Coating.* The normal coating is thin and white. Tongue coating is related to Stomach qi, which, in the process of transforming and digesting food, produces a small amount of unclean residue, or "turbid dampness." This residue flows up to the tongue to form its coating. The presence of a thin coating indicates the normal functioning of digestion. It is also normal for the coating to be slightly thicker on the root than elsewhere on the tongue.

5. *Moisture.* The normal tongue should be slightly moist, neither too dry nor too wet. This again is related to the proper functioning of the Stomach, which is the origin of fluids in the body. When the Stomach functions normally there is a moderate supply of fluids, some of which will reach the tongue.

NOTES

1. For additional information about this topic, see D.W. Beaven and S.E. Brooks, *A Color Atlas of the Tongue in Clinical Diagnosis* (London: Wolfe Medical Publications Ltd., 1988). Illustrations 2-1, 2-2 and 2-3 are based on drawings from this book, adapted and used here with the kind permission of the publisher and the medical illustrator.

TABLE OF ASPECTS OF TONGUE DIAGNOSIS

ASPECT	SPECIFIC FACTOR	CLINICAL SIGNIFICANCE	EIGHT PRINCIPLES DIFFERENTIATION
Tongue spirit		Good or poor prognosis	
Tongue body	Color	Yin Organs, blood, nutritive qi	Cold/hot Yin/yang
	Shape	Yin Organs, blood, qi	Deficiency/excess
Tongue coating	Color	Hot or cold condition	Cold/hot
	Thickness	Strength of pathogenic factor or weakness of body's qi	Deficiency/excess
	Distribution	Exterior conditions: progression of pathogenic factor Interior conditions: location of pathogenic Ta factor	Interior/exterior
	Root	Strength of body's qi, particularly Stomach and Kidney qi	Deficiency/excess
Tongue moisture		Condition of body fluids	Cold/hot Yin/yang

3
Tongue Signs: A Picture of the Internal Organs

One of the principal concepts of Chinese medicine is that there are correspondences among various parts of the body. In pulse diagnosis the pulse on the radial artery can be felt in three sections reflecting the energetic states of the upper, middle and lower parts of the body. In facial diagnosis the face is believed to reflect the condition of different Organs. In tongue diagnosis the same general principle is applied. Certain parts of the tongue reflect the health of other parts of the body, or of certain internal Organs.

This system of correspondences is generally explained by reference to the channels (meridians): a channel originating from an internal Organ reaches the tongue in the course of its pathway; the health of that Organ is reflected on the specific area of the tongue which its channel traverses. Some of the channels (i.e., those of the Lung, Small Intestine, Large Intestine and Gallbladder) do not flow directly to the tongue and yet the health of their associated Organs nonetheless can be reflected there. These channels do, however, indirectly connect with the tongue via their arm-leg related channels (i.e., those of the Spleen, Bladder, Stomach and Triple Burner respectively). All other channels flow directly to the tongue.

The pathways of the channels, however, are at best only a partial explanation. In Chinese medicine there are many phenomena that are attributed to what might be termed a *resonance* between one part of the body and another. This concept can be traced back to the idea of correspondences between macrocosm and microcosm that is an integral part of the five phase theory. In addition to the pulse, face and tongue, the ear, eye, second metacarpal and foot can also reflect and correspond to other parts of the body in ways that cannot be explained by the network of channel pathways alone.

There is thus a complex physiological relationship between the Organs and the tongue. All of the internal Organs connect with the tongue in ways other than via their channels.

Physiologically, the Stomach is the Organ which is most closely related to the tongue: "The tongue coating is the product of the Stomach steaming; the qi of the five yin Organs derives from the Stomach, and therefore one can diagnose the cold or hot and deficient or excess condition of the yin Organs from the tongue coating."[1] In other words, because the tongue coating is a by-product (the "turbid dampness") of the Stomach's digestive activity, and because the Stomach is also the source of qi and blood for all the Organs, it follows that the tongue coating can reflect the condition of all the Organs in terms of heat or cold and excess or deficiency. This is one of the ways in which all of the Organs are physiologically related to the tongue.

Another such relationship between the tongue and the Organs is described in the *Inner Classic:* "The Kidneys control water and receive and store the essence of the five yin Organs and six yang Organs."[2] This means that the Kidneys influence all the other internal Organs by providing them with essence.[3] Since the Kidneys are directly connected to the tongue (the Kidney channel flows to the root of the tongue), and because they supply all the Organs with essence, the health of all the Organs can be reflected in the tongue.

It can therefore be said that all the Organs are physiologically (if somewhat indirectly) related to the tongue via the root of congenital qi (the Kidneys) and the root of acquired qi (the Stomach).[4] The tongue reflects the general state of health of the body, while the specific topography of the tongue reflects the condition of individual Organs.

For diagnostic purposes, there are two major ways of viewing the relationship between the topographical tongue areas and the Organs.

First, the tongue, like the pulse, can be divided into three sections of roughly equal size. The anterior third corresponds to the upper burner, the middle third to the middle burner and the posterior third to the lower burner (ILLUSTRATION 3-1). The Heart and Lungs are situated in the up-

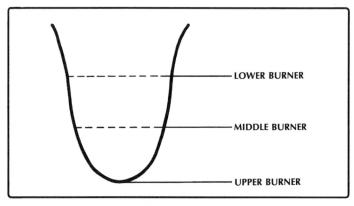

LOWER BURNER

MIDDLE BURNER

UPPER BURNER

Illustration 3-1

per burner, the Stomach and Spleen are in the middle burner and the Bladder, Kidneys, Small Intestine and Large Intestine are in the lower burner. (For a more thorough discussion of the three burners differentiation, SEE APPENDIX III.)

As often happens in Chinese medicine, functional relationships are more important than structural ones. The assignment of internal Organs to the three burners reflects the functional relationships of the Organs to particular burners,

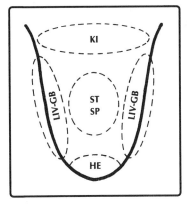

Illustration 3-2

rather than the anatomical relationship of the Organs to those particular zones of the body. This explains why the Liver is sometimes regarded as part of the lower burner (since so many of its related pathological conditions are reflected there) and sometimes as part of the middle burner. Similarly, the Gallbladder is not usually mentioned as part of the middle burner simply because the middle burner is a generalization which indicates the digestive functions of the Spleen and Stomach.

There are various systems which describe the correspondences between specific areas of the tongue and individual Organs, but the differences among them are not great. Two examples will suffice (ILLUSTRATIONS 3-2 & 3-3).

The tip of the tongue corresponds to the Heart, the center to the Stomach and Spleen, the sides to the Liver and Gallbladder and the root to the Kidneys.[5]

The root of the tongue corresponds to the Kidneys, gate of vitality *(ming mén),* Large Intestine, Small Intestine and Bladder; the center-left to the Stomach; the center-right to the Spleen; the area between the center and the tip to the Lungs; the tip to the Heart and Pericardium; the left side to the Liver; and the right edge to the Gallbladder.[6]

The second passage above probably represents the most common scheme of tongue topography, except in two details. The correspondence of the Stomach with the center-left and the Spleen with the center-right of the tongue is not widely used. Instead, it is said that the center of the tongue corresponds to the Stomach and the area immediately around the center to the Spleen.[7] The author finds this to be true in clinical practice. The tongue area correspondences used in this book (ILLUSTRATION 3-4) will therefore be the following: the tongue tip corresponds to the Heart; the area between the tip and center to the Lungs; the center to the Stomach and Spleen; the root to the Kidneys, Intestines and Bladder (and, in women, to the Womb); the left edge to the Liver; and the right edge to the Gallbladder.

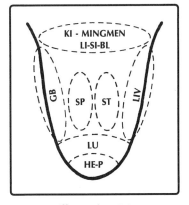

Illustration 3-3

A second method of observing the relationship between the topography of the tongue and the Organs is through the papillae. As we have seen, the papillae of the tongue are, from a modern biomedical perspective, small projections in the mucous membrane which cover the dorsum of the tongue. Five types of papillae are recognized: foliate, filiform, fungiform, vallate and circumvallate. Ancient Chinese writings recognized only two types of papillae and, typically for Chinese medicine, saw a functional relationship between them and some of the internal Organs. Illustrative of this approach is the following passage from *Simple Study of Diagnosis from Body Forms and Facial Color:*

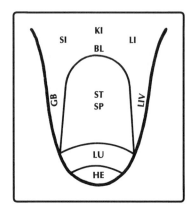

If the tip of the tongue has fine red grains, it indicates that Heart qi holds the true fire of the gate of vitality[8] as it arises; if the center of the tongue has white soft prickles as fine as hair, it indicates that Lung qi holds the true fire of the gate of vitality as it comes out.[9]

From the classical Chinese perspective, when the physiological fire of the gate of vitality joins up with the Heart, the tip of the tongue will have pale red papillae; when it joins up with the Lungs, the center of the tongue will have soft white papillae. A healthy, pale red tip and soft white center therefore indicates health in the Heart, Lungs and Kidneys (because the gate of vitality is related to Kidney yang).

Illustration 3-4

NOTES

1. Zhou Xue-Hai, *Simple Study of Diagnosis from Body Forms and Facial Color (Xing se wai zhen jian mo)* (1894). Cited in Beijing College of Traditional Chinese Medicine, *Tongue Diagnosis in Chinese Medicine (Zhong yi she zhen)* (Beijing: People's Medical Publishing House, 1976), p. 8.

2. *Yellow Emperor's Inner Classic: Simple Questions (Huang di nei jing su wen)* (Beijing: People's Medical Publishing House, 1963), p. 6.

3. The essence *(jing)* is partly inherited from the parents and determines our constitution and potential for biological development. The essence is stored in the Kidneys.

4. The congenital qi, literally "pre-heaven qi" *(xian tian zhi qi)*, indicates the basic constitution of a human being and is another term for the essence received from the parents and stored in the Kidneys. It is called congenital because it is formed before birth. Acquired qi, literally "post-heaven qi" *(hou tian zhi qi)*, refers to the qi and blood formed by the activities of the Spleen and Stomach after birth. Because the Kidneys store essence and the Spleen and Stomach produce the qi after birth, they are called the root of congenital qi and the root of acquired qi, respectively.

5. Jian Bi-Hua, *Mirror of Medicine (Yi jing)* (1641). Cited in *Tongue Diagnosis in Chinese Medicine*, p. 8.

6. Lian Te-Yan, *Differentiation of Syndromes by Examination of the Tongue (She jian bian zheng)* (1906). Cited in *Tongue Diagnosis in Chinese Medicine*, p. 8.

7. Guangdong College of Traditional Medicine, *Chinese Medical Diagnosis (Zhong yi zhen duan xue)* (Shanghai: Shanghai Scientific Publishing House, 6th edition, 1979), p. 14.

8. The concept of the gate of vitality *(ming men)* has occupied Chinese physicians for centuries. The main sources of information concerning this concept are the *Classic of Difficulties, Thousand Ducat Prescriptions* and *Medical Treasury (Yi gui),* the latter written in 1687 by Zhao Xian-He. There have been countless discussions concerning whether the gate of vitality corresponds to the right Kidney (as in chapter 36 of *Classic of Difficulties)* or is situated between the two Kidneys (as in chapter 66 of *Classic of Difficulties,* and in *Medical Treasury).* Basically, the gate of vitality corresponds to the fire within the Kidneys. It is a physiological fire (hence called the "true fire of the gate of vitality") which has the functions of warming the Heart to assist it in housing spirit, warming the Stomach and Spleen to assist their function of digestion, and warming the Bladder and lower burner to assist their function of transformation and excretion of fluids. When the gate of vitality's fire declines, the Heart suffers, the Stomach and Spleen cannot digest food, the Bladder and lower burner cannot transform fluids, the essence of the Kidneys turns cold and the uterus becomes weak and cold, causing infertility or chronic leukorrhea. Some modern textbooks have simplified the concept of the gate of vitality by regarding it as no more than a different expression for Kidney yang. They reason that because Kidney yin is the material substratum of Kidney yang, the two cannot be clearly distinguished. The gate of vitality thus serves to denote the outward manifestations of Kidney yang, and its effect is clearly manifested in pathological conditions such as the decline of physiological fire.

9. *Simple Study of Diagnosis from Body Forms and Facial Color.* Cited in *Tongue Diagnosis in Chinese Medicine,* p. 7.

4
The Eight Principles in Tongue Diagnosis

The identification of disease patterns according to the eight principles is perhaps the cardinal method in Chinese medicine for analyzing the pathogenesis of disease and rationally interpreting the types of disharmony that result. Examination of the tongue is a very important part of this method. As mentioned in chapter 3, the tongue body color is one of the pillars of diagnosis, and is particularly important in differentiating patterns according to the eight principles. The tongue coating is also important, especially in differentiating exterior from interior and hot from cold patterns.

In order to relate tongue diagnosis to the eight principles, our discussion will focus on the most common types of tongues to be found in each of the eight categories, i.e., exterior/interior, hot/cold, excess/deficiency and yin/yang. This approach is, in a sense, contradictory to the very spirit of Chinese diagnosis, which involves the integration of the findings from all of the four traditional methods of diagnosis. Furthermore, just as the four methods of diagnosis must be integrated, so too must all of the categories of the eight principles identification of patterns be viewed as a whole. This makes generalization difficult. For example, how the tongue will appear in the presence of an exterior pattern will depend on whether this is excessive or deficient, cold or hot. Nevertheless, it is still useful to describe the tongue signs in each of the eight categories to grasp their essential characteristics, with the understanding that the actual signs in clinical practice will be more complex.

EXTERIOR

An exterior condition is characterized by invasion of an external pathogenic factor (cold, dampness, heat, dryness or wind) in the exterior layers of the body (skin, muscles, channels or sinews). When such invasion occurs, the patient is said to display exterior symptoms and signs.

Generally speaking, an external attack will not produce discernible changes on the tongue in the initial stages. For example, in an attack from external wind-cold the tongue coating is said to be thin and white. However, a thin white coating is also normal, and in many cases of mild wind-cold attack the tongue coating will not change significantly.

The pathogenic factors of heat and cold are almost always associated with wind and will accordingly be discussed in conjunction with wind in the analyses which follow. Wind is the most dynamic of the pathogenic factors, and the one that usually combines itself with the others. Other pathogenic factors may be said to "ride" the wind in order to penetrate the exterior layers of the body.

Wind-Cold

In the initial stages of an attack by wind-cold the tongue coating will be thin, white and probably overly moist. The coating is white because of the cold, thin because the pathogenic factor is in the initial stages and therefore not too strong, and overly moist because the cold in the exterior layers blocks the proper movement of body fluids in the skin and muscles, leading to a slight accumulation of fluids. In its initial stages, this coating from attack of wind-cold frequently appears only in the front part of the tongue between the tip and the center. This coating can be scraped off (because the pathogenic factor is still mild) but will soon return as long as the pathogenic factor is present.

If the whole coating is white and dry and cannot be scraped off, it indicates that the externally-contracted cold is about to penetrate deeper and has the potential of turning into fire, which would make the tongue dry. In this case, the coating covers the entire tongue.

If in the initial stages of an attack of wind-cold the coating is thin white with dry prickles, this indicates that the cold is about to transform into heat and that the Lung fluids have been injured, resulting in the dry prickles.

If the coating is thin white and greasy, the presence of externally-contracted damp-cold, in the initial stage of penetration, is indicated. The greasy coating is a sign that dampness is present.

Wind-Heat

In the initial stages of an attack by wind-heat the tongue coating will be thin, white and dry. It is thin because the pathogenic factor is just entering the body, white because it is at the initial stage and has not yet produced much heat within the body, and dry because wind-heat dries up the body fluids. As the heat starts to penetrate, the tongue coating will be thin and yellow. In severe cases of attack by wind-heat the tongue coating may also be gray or black and have prickles rising out of its surface.

Frequently, in attacks by wind-heat only the front part of the tongue will display changes in the coating. The tongue body may also manifest changes with the front and edges turning red. This should not be confused with a situation of Heart fire or Liver fire. Aside from other very different clinical signs and symptoms, an attack by wind-heat usually causes the entire front part of the tongue to become red, while in cases of Heart fire only the very tip will do so.

In children, exterior invasions of wind-heat often manifest with red points in the front and/or sides (PLATE 41).

INTERIOR

An interior condition is characterized by the presence of a pathogenic factor in the interior of the body. The pathogenic factor could be internal dampness, wind, fire, dryness or cold, or it could simply be an internal imbalance between yin and yang. There could, for example, be the presence of Liver fire, a real pathogenic factor, or merely an imbalance between Kidney yin and Liver yang. The chief characteristic of an interior disease is its residence in the internal Organs, as opposed to the exterior portions of the body (skin, muscles, sinews and channels). It is practically impossible to generalize about the appearance of the tongue in an interior condition because there are so many different possible pathological situations.

The tongue topography can reflect the evolution of disease from the exterior to the interior or vice versa (see chapter 3). However, the word "evolution" must be stressed here. Tongue topography should not be interpreted in a rigid way, with a fixed system of correspondence between tongue areas and body parts. The same area of the tongue may reflect the status of different body parts under different conditions. It is essential to integrate the findings of tongue diagnosis with those of other diagnostic methods. Furthermore, the correspondence of tongue areas to body parts is sometimes only apparent over the course of a disease, as the location of the pathogenic factor changes.

With those reservations in mind, as a general rule the perimeters of the tongue correspond to the exterior of the body, and the central areas to the interior (ILLUSTRATION 4-1).

Movement between exterior and interior can be reflected on the tongue as movement from the tip to the root, the tip corresponding to the exterior and the root to the interior of the body. This interpretation is compatible with the notion that the three-part division of the tongue, anterior to posterior,

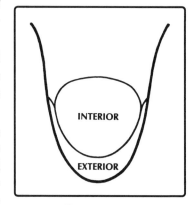

Illustration 4-1

corresponds to the three burners: upper, middle and lower. The anterior part of the tongue generally corresponds to the exterior, and the posterior part to the interior (ILLUSTRATION 4-2). Integrating these interpretations, one could say that the

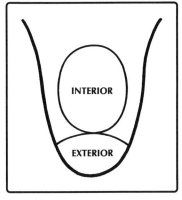

Illustration 4-2

upper burner is more "exterior" than the middle or lower burners. This does not mean that all upper burner diseases are external in origin. It does mean that the Lungs, which are situated in the upper burner and control the skin and the protective qi, correspond to the exterior, to which the anterior part of the tongue also corresponds.

It is generally said that the tongue coating is yellow in interior conditions. This is only partly true since a yellow coating indicates heat, and there may well be interior conditions characterized by cold, in which case the coating would be white. However, an interior condition either develops from an exterior one or develops independently, usually with slow progress over a long period of time. One can therefore say that the coating would *usually* be yellow because pathogenic factors tend to transform into heat once inside the body for a long time.

One can also generally say that when the coating turns from white to yellow the disease has penetrated to the interior. In some cases the tongue coating could also be partially white and partially yellow. If the coating is white around the edges and yellow at the central surface of the tongue, it indicates that the pathogenic factor has penetrated into the interior and transformed into heat. This is so because the outside of the tongue corresponds to the exterior of the body and the center corresponds to the interior. Similarly, if the coating is yellow on the edges and white in the center, it indicates that the pathogenic factor is losing its strength and the condition is improving. Finally, the absence of coating altogether is always indicative of an interior condition, usually of Stomach and Kidney yin deficiency.

HALF-INTERIOR, HALF-EXTERIOR CONDITIONS

Those conditions described in Chinese medicine as "half-interior, half-exterior" involve location of the pathogenic factor at a level between the interior and exterior portions of the body. A half-interior, half-exterior disease is also called a lesser yang disease and is characterized by alternating chills and fever, a bitter taste in the mouth, hypochondriac pain, irritability, dry throat and nausea. The tongue coating in this case is typically white and slightly slippery and is located only on the right side (ILLUSTRATION 4-3a). There are, however,

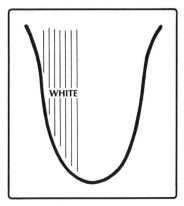

Illustration 4-3a

other types and distributions of tongue coating which indicate the presence of a half-interior, half-exterior disease: a red tongue body with white coating

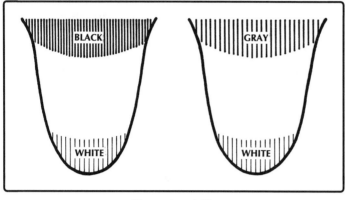

Illustration 4-3b

on the tip only; a white coating on the tip and black coating on the root; and a white coating on the tip and gray coating on the root (ILLUSTRATION 4-3b).

COLD

Cold is manifested both in the tongue body and the tongue body coating. The tongue body will be pale and the coating white and overly moist. There is a distinction between deficiency cold and excess cold.

Deficiency Cold

A deficiency cold condition arises from deficiency of yang qi. In this situation the tongue body will be pale and the coating thin, white and overly moist. The tongue body is pale because the deficient yang qi fails to carry qi and blood to the tongue. The coating is thin because the condition arises from deficiency; there is no actual pathogenic factor in the body to show on the tongue coating. It is white because of the cold and overly moist because the deficient yang qi fails to transform and transport the fluids throughout the body, which then accumulate on the tongue.

In less common cases of very severe and long-standing deficiency of yang, the tongue may also be dry instead of overly moist. This occurs because the yang qi is so deficient that it fails to transport fluids at all.

Excess Cold

Conditions arising from an excess of yin or cold can either be exterior or interior. The exterior form, as in wind-cold, has already been discussed above.

Interior excess cold is manifested on the tongue by a pale body and a thick, white coating which is overly moist and possibly slippery. The tongue body is pale because the excess cold obstructs the circulation of yang qi, which is then unable to carry blood to the tongue. The coating is thick; thickness of coating is one of the primary characteristics which distinguishes excess cold from deficiency cold. The coating is also white and overly moist or slippery. When excess cold obstructs the circulation of yang qi, the latter fails to transform and transport the fluids, which then accumulate on the tongue.

In both deficiency cold and excess cold conditions the tongue body can also be blue. This usually occurs when there is chronic retention of cold.

Finally, cold can be indicated by a purple-blue tongue body. This appears in cases of prolonged cold retention when circulation is obstructed and stasis of blood occurs.

HEAT

In heat conditions the tongue body is either red or dark red. In excess heat conditions the coating will be yellow, while in deficiency heat conditions there will be no coating at all. In both cases the tongue will be dry. In general, the darker the tongue body and the darker yellow the coating, the more heat there is.

Heat will be manifested in different ways depending upon its point of concentration in the body. Heart heat is indicated by a red tongue tip with red points. Liver heat is manifested by red sides and bilateral yellow coating. Stomach heat is indicated by a thick yellow coating, often with red points around the center of the tongue. Lung heat often appears as a thin yellow coating on the anterior of the tongue. In all of these cases the tongue will be dry. Brown, gray and black coatings may also indicate the presence of heat, in a degree more serious than is indicated by a yellow coating. Coatings that are dry and brown or black are often seen in cases of extreme heat in the Stomach and Intestines, with retention of desiccated feces.

DEFICIENCY

A condition of deficiency is characterized by an insufficiency of the body's energies. Deficiencies of qi, yang, blood and yin each have their distinctive expressions in the tongue.

Qi Deficiency

In deficient qi conditions the tongue body may be slightly flabby without any other signs. The tongue body may even appear normal if the deficiency is not very severe. The tongue appearance in qi deficiency will vary according to which Organ is most affected.

LUNG QI DEFICIENCY

The Lungs control qi and respiration. Together with the Spleen, it is the Organ most often affected by deficiency of qi. The pathological signs include shortness of breath, weak voice and spontaneous sweating. If the Lung qi deficiency is not too severe, the tongue body may not show it. In long-standing deficiency it might be slightly swollen in the anterior part between tip and center. This would be the only sign of Lung qi deficiency as the tongue body color is normal or slightly pale and there are no other abnormalities. Sometimes the Lung area (between the tip and center of the tongue) has a thin white coating which is also slightly moist. This indicates retention of cold in the Lungs from a previous attack of wind-cold that was not properly treated.

SPLEEN QI DEFICIENCY

The Spleen controls the physiological activities of transformation and transportation of fluids and food essence. It is an Organ easily affected by qi deficiency, the main manifestations of which are lethargy, poor appetite, and abdominal distension. The tongue will be tooth-marked, slightly swollen and possibly pale, even though there are no symptoms of cold. If the condition is very slight, there may be no manifestations on the tongue at all.

STOMACH QI DEFICIENCY

The Stomach transforms and separates the food from fluids. A small amount of "turbid dampness" left over from this process flows up to the tongue and forms the coating. A thin white coating is normal and indicates proper functioning of the Stomach. In Stomach qi deficiency the digestive process is impaired and as a result no turbid dampness is transported to the tongue. This condition is indicated by either a thinning of the coating in the center of the tongue, or a coating without root.

HEART QI DEFICIENCY

The Heart controls the blood and blood vessels. A deficiency of Heart qi will be manifested in circulatory irregularities, causing palpitations and shortness of breath during exertion. The tongue body will be pale (even though there are no symptoms of cold) because the deficient Heart qi fails to carry blood to it. In more severe cases of Heart qi deficiency, the tip of the tongue will be slightly swollen while the body will be pale. This is often the result of emotional trauma, which disperses Heart qi.

Yang Deficiency

In Yang deficiency the tongue body will be pale because the deficient yang qi fails to carry blood to it. It will also be overly wet because the fluids which deficient yang qi fails to transform and transport throughout the body accumulate on the tongue. The coating will be thin because of the deficiency condition, and white because of the cold induced by insufficient yang qi.

The appearance of the tongue in this situation will vary according to which Organ is most affected.

SPLEEN YANG DEFICIENCY

The Spleen is easily affected by yang deficiency, often caused by the excessive consumption of cold or raw foods. The clinical manifestations are similar to those of Spleen qi deficiency described above, with the addition of chilliness and very loose stool. The tongue will definitely be pale, or very pale and possibly somewhat swollen, since the deficiency of Spleen yang may lead to the accumulation of dampness. The tongue will also be overly wet and the coating will be white. If there is dampness the tongue will be rather swollen, but otherwise not.

KIDNEY YANG DEFICIENCY

Kidney yang deficiency often accompanies Spleen yang deficiency and always indicates a more severe condition. It exhibits the clinical signs of Spleen yang deficiency, but in addition there will be soreness of the back, chilliness, dizziness, very loose stool in the early morning and great lassitude. The tongue will be very pale, swollen and overly wet; the coating will be white. The appearance of the tongue in Spleen yang and Kidney yang deficiency is basically the same; they cannot be easily distinguished except that sometimes in Kidney yang deficiency the tongue will be wetter and paler than in Spleen yang deficiency. Reference must be made to other clinical manifestations.

HEART YANG DEFICIENCY

The clinical signs of Heart yang deficiency are the same as those of Heart qi deficiency, with the addition of chilliness, cold hands and a bright white facial pallor. The tongue will be pale and its tip may possibly be paler or slightly more moist than the rest of the tongue. In severe and persistent cases of Heart yang deficiency there is stasis of blood in the chest, resulting in chest pains and cyanosis of the lips. In this situation the tongue will be bluish-purple (a pale tongue turned purple). Stasis of blood in the Heart will be indicated by purple spots on the sides between the center and tip of the tongue (ILLUSTRATION 4-4).

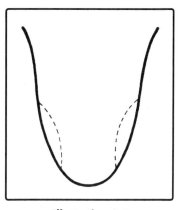

Illustration 4-4

Blood Deficiency

In Blood Deficiency the tongue body will be pale and slightly dry. Blood and fluids have the same origin. Thus the deficiency which causes the tongue to be pale for lack of blood also causes its relative dryness, as less fluid reaches the tongue.

Once again, the appearance of the tongue in conditions of blood deficiency will vary according to which Organ is most affected. Spleen blood deficiency and Liver blood deficiency are the most common patterns.

SPLEEN BLOOD DEFICIENCY

The Spleen is the origin of blood which is produced from the essence which the Spleen extracts from food. A deficiency in the Spleen's transformation of food will often lead to a general deficiency of blood. The tongue will be pale and dry. If Spleen blood deficiency is accompanied by Heart blood deficiency the tip of the tongue will be paler still. Clinical signs of Spleen blood deficiency include numbness, tiredness, a pale face and dizziness. If accompanied by Heart blood deficiency there will also be insomnia and palpitations.

LIVER BLOOD DEFICIENCY

Any deficiency of blood may affect the Liver because the Liver stores blood. Liver blood deficiency is indicated when the sides are paler than the rest of the tongue. In severe and persistent cases, especially when the condition has become deficient yin, the sides of the tongue may even have an orange hue.

Clinical manifestations include dizziness and numbness, a pale face, brittle nails and, in women, scanty periods.

Yin Deficiency

Deficiency of yin implies depletion of the vital essences, the nutrient substances of the body. It is therefore the most serious variety of deficiency. It usually arises in chronic conditions after a long time due to irregular diet, overwork and/or excessive sexual activity. This condition can also occur in acute cases as a consequence of externally-contracted heat burning up the body's fluids. This happens, for example, in poliomyelitis when high temperature is followed by a paralysis due to the withering of muscles and sinews from heat's exhaustion of yin fluids.

In chronic cases, the Organs most affected by yin deficiency are the Stomach, Lungs, Heart and Kidneys. Since deficiency leads to an exhaustion of fluids which cool the body, fire can predominate and run out of control. This condition of yin deficiency complicated by fire excess is called fire or heat from deficiency, also known as "empty fire" or "empty heat". It almost always causes the tongue to become red or dark red. Since the Stomach is the origin of fluids in the body, a deficiency of Stomach yin is often the first stage of a general yin deficiency. The tongue will be peeled, i.e., will have no coating at all, or will have a coating without root. The lack of yin fluids resulting from yin deficiency will make the tongue dry.

STOMACH YIN DEFICIENCY

Stomach yin deficiency is often the first stage of general yin deficiency; there is no deficiency heat and the tongue is not red. The tongue may have a coating without root because the deficient Stomach yin fails to produce new coating matter, while the old coating becomes rootless. After this stage, there occurs a complete absence of coating on the central surface of the tongue. The clinical signs of Stomach yin deficiency may vary but usually there is dryness in the mouth and throat, epigastric pain, thirst possibly accompanied by an inability to drink, or a desire to drink warm water or to drink in small sips, loss of appetite and dry stool.

KIDNEY YIN DEFICIENCY

Kidney yin deficiency often represents a more advanced stage of Stomach yin deficiency in the course of a chronic condition. Kidney yin deficiency is often followed by the arousal of pathological minister fire, since control of fire by the yin fluids is lacking. This is fire or deficiency heat which, when severe, can also be called "reckless fire." Because of the presence of heat from yin deficiency, the tongue will be red or dark red, dry and peeled (completely without coating).

Frequently, the tongue will also have a deep crack in the midline that reaches the tip. The deeper this crack, the more severe and established is the Kidney yin deficiency. Other clinical manifestations can be manifold but usually include tinnitus, vertigo, deafness, soreness of the back, afternoon and evening feverishness, dry mouth during the night, dryness of the throat, nocturnal emissions, night sweats, insomnia and impaired memory.

HEART YIN DEFICIENCY

Heart yin deficiency almost always derives from Kidney yin deficiency. The tongue will be red, peeled and dry. In addition, the tip may be redder and drier than the rest of the tongue, indicating the arousal of pathological minister fire from deficiency in the Heart. Clinical signs will be similar to those of Kidney yin deficiency, with the addition of insomnia, mental restlessness and palpitations.

LUNG YIN DEFICIENCY

Lung yin deficiency may either lead to, or be a consequence of, Kidney yin deficiency. Typical clinical manifestations include sweating of the sternal area, palms and soles of the feet (called "heat in the five centers" or "five-palm heat"); afternoon and evening feverishness; dryness of the throat; and a weak cough with scanty sputum that may be tinged with blood. The tongue will be red, peeled and dry, and may have one or two cracks in its Lung area.

EXCESS

A condition of excess is one in which the body's energies are still vital and reacting to the pathogenic factors, whether they are in the exterior or interior levels of the body. The symptoms and signs of an excessive condition are therefore characterized by the struggle between the body's energies and the pathogenic energies. The signs occur in a sudden fashion, and include restlessness and acute changes in temperature, among other symptoms.

It is difficult to generalize about what the tongue looks like in excessive conditions since this depends on whether the condition is one of heat or cold, of the exterior or interior, or of yin or yang. However, there are a few characteristic features of excessive conditions.

First of all, the tongue body color is usually not pale; paleness indicates deficiency of blood or yang. The exception to this is cold, which can also lead to a pale tongue. A condition of excess can, however, coexist with one of deficiency. It is possible to have a yang qi deficiency (indicated by a pale tongue) with an excess of dampness in the body (with a consequent swollen and wet tongue).

The coating provides a better indication of excess or deficiency. A thick coating usually indicates the presence of a pathogenic factor, and therefore a condition of excess. A thin or rootless coating, or the complete absence of coating, indicates weakness and exhaustion of the body's energies, i.e., a condition of deficiency. The consistency of the tongue body can also be used to distinguish between excess and deficiency. A stiff tongue body indicates excess, while a flabby one is a sign of deficiency. A swollen body usually indicates an excessive condition (retention of dampness or phlegm) while a thin body indicates a condition of deficiency (blood or yin deficiency).

Exterior Excess

Exterior excess conditions involve an attack of external cold or heat, previously discussed in this chapter.

Interior Excess

This category includes conditions of interior excess cold, interior excess heat, blood stasis and phlegm.

INTERIOR EXCESS COLD

Interior excess cold conditions involve an accumulation of cold in the Organs. Examples of this type of condition include the presence of dampness in the Spleen and retention of cold in the Intestines, Womb or chest. In such conditions, the tongue body is pale because of the cold. The coating is white and usually thick. The tongue body might also be blue or bluish purple, indicating a severe and persistent retention of cold in the body, with subsequent stagnation.

INTERIOR EXCESS HEAT

Interior excess heat conditions are characterized by the presence of fire in the body. Examples include fire in the Heart, blazing Liver fire, Lung heat and Stomach fire. The tongue body will always be red or dark red, and the coating will be yellow and usually thick. (In excess heat there is a coating, while in deficiency heat there is little or no coating.)

BLOOD STASIS

Stasis of blood is always an excessive condition, even though it may be caused by a deficient condition such as qi or blood deficiency. The clinical signs vary with the location of the disorder. In general, blood stasis is accompanied by persistent, localized pain which may be of a stabbing, boring or pricking nature. If there is bleeding, the blood will be scanty and dark purple. Any pressure will aggravate the pain. The tongue, a very reliable indicator of blood stasis, will be purple in color and have dark red or purple spots.

The location of the purple spots on the tongue can identify the physical locus of the condition. Spots on the sides of the tongue in the area between tip and center (ILLUSTRATION 4-5) mean stasis of blood in the chest, with accompanying angina-like pain.

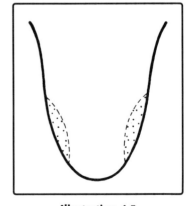

Illustration 4-5

Spots all along the sides of the tongue mean stasis of blood in the Liver. If the purple spots are on the central surface of the tongue, blood stasis in the Stomach is indicated. If the spots are on the root, it is a sign of stasis of blood in the Intestines or Bladder. Blood stasis can also manifest on the underside of the tongue as swelling and darkening of the two veins on either side of the frenulum.

PHLEGM

Phlegm is always an excessive condition in itself, even though it is usually caused by a deficiency condition. When Spleen yang, Kidney yang and, to a certain extent, Lung qi are deficient, the fluids cannot be transformed and transported. After a long time the fluids may congeal, become more yin and give rise to phlegm. The clinical manifestations of phlegm vary widely depending on the location of the condition and the nature of the phlegm, whether substantial or insubstantial. In general, a thick, slippery and greasy coating on the tongue always indicates the presence of phlegm.

SUMMARY

Careful analysis of the tongue body color and shape and tongue coating color, thickness and distribution can provide a clear reflection of the character of the disease pattern from the perspective of the eight principles:

- For exterior conditions, look at the coating. Its distribution in the front part or around the center confirms an exterior condition. Its thickness gives an indication of the strength of the external pathogenic factor (the thicker the coating, the stronger the pathogenic factor).
- For interior conditions, look at the tongue body. Its color and shape will clearly reflect the presence of any internal disharmony.
- For cold conditions, look at the tongue body color (pale) and coating (white).
- For conditions of heat, look at the tongue body color (red) and coating (yellow).
- For conditions of excess, look at the tongue body shape (swollen, stiff) and coating thickness (thick).
- For conditions of deficiency, look at the tongue body color (pale in yang and blood deficiency, red in yin deficiency), the tongue body shape (flaccid, thin) and the coating (none or rootless).

TABLE OF THE EIGHT PRINCIPLES DIFFERENTIATION

CONDITION	SPECIFIC FACTOR	TONGUE SIGNS
Exterior		Wind cold: coating thin and white Wind heat: coating thin and white in the initial stage, then yellow
Interior		Tongue body color and shape altered
Half-interior, half-exterior		White coating on one side only, or white anteriorly, gray or black posteriorly
Cold		Coating white Deficiency: body pale
Hot		Body red, coating yellow
Deficiency	Qi	Lung: body slightly flaccid, slightly swollen anteriorly Spleen: tooth-marked Stomach: lack of coating in the center Heart: body pale
	Yang	Body pale Spleen: body pale, coating white, wet Kidney: body pale and swollen, coating white Heart: body pale, bluish purple if severe
	Blood	Spleen: body pale, slightly dry Heart: body pale, tip paler Liver: body pale, sides paler
	Yin	Stomach: no coating in center, dry, wide crack in the center Kidney: body red, no coating, dry, cracks Heart: body red, no coating anteriorly, tip redder Lungs: body red, no coating, cracks anteriorly
Excess	Exterior	Coating thick
	Interior	Cold: body pale, coating thick, slippery and white Hot: body red, coating thick and yellow Stasis of blood: body purple Phlegm: coating thick, slippery and greasy

5
Tongue Spirit and Body Color

When examining the tongue, five primary aspects must be considered. These are the tongue spirit, tongue body color, tongue body shape (including its consistency and mobility), tongue coating, and tongue moisture. In this and the following two chapters, each of these aspects will be discussed in turn.

TONGUE SPIRIT

Despite its name, this aspect of the tongue has no metaphysical significance. "Spirit" in this context denotes an indefinable appearance associated with health and vitality. The Chinese word, *shén,* also has the meaning of "look" or "expression." The characteristic of having or not having *shén* applies to other elements of diagnosis as well, including the eyes, the complexion and the pulse.

A tongue is said to have spirit when it appears to be flourishing and robust, and no spirit when it appears to be withered. Flourishing means possessing vitality and brightness. Even in disease a tongue with these attributes indicates a condition that is easily cured (PLATES 1 & 17). A tongue lacking vitality and brightness (i.e., without spirit) indicates that the disease will be difficult to cure (PLATES 13, 23 & 27).

The quality of spirit is described in *A Guide to Tongue Differentiation:*

A flourishing and moist tongue indicates a good supply of body fluids. A dry and withered tongue indicates the exhaustion of body fluids. Flourishing is called 'to have spirit' and indicates brightness, clear color, freshness and a light red color. All these attributes indicate life; the absence of them indicates death. A bright, moist and blood-colored tongue indicates life; a dark, withered tongue with no blood color indicates death.[1]

One can thus distinguish a "life" tongue from a "death" tongue. The life tongue displays a lively red color on the root. The death tongue displays a dark color on the root and is withered. The root of the tongue reflects the health of the

Kidneys, which store the essence. Healthy essence (manifested in a lively red color of the root) is conducive to a healthy life, while deficient essence (manifested in a dark color and withered appearance of the root) leads to ill health and death. Although this distinction cannot be taken literally (a death tongue does not necessarily imply imminent death in all cases), it is still useful as a distinguishing characteristic of mild or serious conditions.

The tongue spirit is also a useful tool in prognosis. The presence of spirit in the tongue indicates a good prognosis, even if the tongue is pathological in other respects. Plate 28, a tongue of a 93 year-old woman, is a good example of this principle: although it has a very thick, dry, black coating (indicating fire in the Intestines), the tongue body (more visible on the sides) nevertheless does have spirit.

TONGUE BODY COLOR

Tongue body color is the color of the tongue itself, beneath its coating. It is the single most important aspect of tongue diagnosis. Tongue body color almost always reflects the true condition of the body since it is unaffected by secondary and short-term factors.

To reiterate what was said in chapter 2, the normal tongue body color is pale and red, and the tongue itself is moist. It is red because there is a sufficient supply of blood from the Heart to the tongue, and the yang qi moves freely, pushing the blood to the tongue. It is pale because there is a sufficient supply of fluids reaching the tongue from the Stomach, the origin of fluids in the body. In the words of one traditional medical text, "The tongue is the offshoot of the Heart, hence its color is red; its body is moist; its surface is as thin as hair without thorns; its coating is thin and white."[2]

The clinical significance of the tongue body color is that it reflects the health of the Organs, blood, and nutritive qi. From the perspective of patterns identification, it reflects the hot and cold influences, yin and yang and stagnation of qi or blood.

The tongue body colors that will be considered are pale, red, dark red, purple and blue. Red here indicates a color which is redder than the normal pale red.

Pale

A pale tongue body color includes shades from slightly paler than normal to nearly white, in extreme cases. The paler the tongue body color, the more serious the condition. The degree of paleness can be used as a gauge for prognosis.

In clinical practice two situations can arise in connection with a pale tongue: either the blood itself is deficient, or yang qi is deficient and fails to supply the tongue with blood. If the condition results from yang deficiency there will also be symptoms of interior cold. If there is blood deficiency the tongue will tend to be dry. If there is yang deficiency it will tend to be overly wet.

In women, blood deficiency is the more common cause of a pale tongue, while in men yang deficiency is more common. In men, a pale tongue will hardly ever be caused by deficient blood, but among women there is a significant, although less common, incidence of a pale tongue due to deficient yang (PLATE 9).

Other clinical manifestations of deficient blood include numbness, dizziness, impaired memory, a dull, pale face, insomnia, scanty periods in women and a choppy pulse. Other clinical manifestations of deficient yang include chilliness, loose stool, a bright, white face and a deep, weak pulse.

PALE WET

By "wet" here is meant that fluid is clearly visible on the surface of the tongue. In extreme cases the tongue may be wet to the point of dripping saliva.

A pale wet tongue indicates deficiency of Spleen yang, which fails to transform and transport fluids, causing their accumulation on the tongue. The deficient yang qi also fails to "push" blood to the tongue, which then becomes pale.

A pale wet tongue can also indicate Kidney yang deficiency, in which case the tongue would also be swollen. A chronic Spleen yang deficiency can easily lead to Kidney yang deficiency, aggravating the condition (PLATE 9).

Clinical manifestations of Spleen yang deficiency with a pale wet tongue include lack of appetite, abdominal distension, lassitude, a bright, white complexion, loose stool, coldness in the limbs, chilliness and a deep, weak pulse. This condition is particularly common in young people, and especially in women. It is often due to excessive consumption of cold and raw foods and iced drinks.

One type of pale wet tongue is accompanied by a sticky coating. A pale, very swollen tongue body with a sticky coating all over may indicate obstruction of the spirit by phlegm, which may manifest in severe anxiety or mildly manic behavior (PLATES 45 & 46).

PALE DRY

A pale dry tongue usually indicates blood deficiency. Blood and fluids are so closely related that an insufficiency of one often leads to an insufficiency of the other. They are both part of the yin of the body. When blood is deficient not enough blood or fluids reach the tongue, which becomes pale and dry.

A pale dry tongue can also indicate a completely different pattern. Fluids originate in the Stomach from the transformation of food and drink by yang qi, which also distributes the fluids throughout the body. This is a function particularly of Lung qi, Spleen yang and Kidney yang. If both the Lung qi and Spleen yang are deficient, the Stomach cannot generate the fluids, the Spleen cannot transform and transport them and the Lung qi cannot disperse them. When the fluids cannot reach the tongue it becomes dry. In this case the dryness of the tongue is not due to deficient blood, but to deficient yang.

Thus deficiency of yang qi can be indicated by either a wet or a dry tongue, although the former is much more common. Other clinical signs must also be taken into account. In the former case the tongue is wet because the accumulating fluids are not transformed and transported by Spleen yang. In the latter case the tongue is dry because the fluids are not generated in the Stomach, are not dispersed by Lung qi, and do not reach the tongue. It cannot be inferred from the evidence of the pale dry tongue alone whether the condition is due to blood deficiency or yang deficiency. Yang deficiency with a dry tongue is more serious than the same pattern with a wet tongue (PLATE 6).

In addition to a pale dry tongue, other clinical manifestations of blood deficiency include pale complexion, numb sensations, dizziness, impaired memory, insomnia, pale lips, scanty periods in women and a choppy pulse. This condition is extremely common among women. In severe cases it can lead to infertility since an abundant supply of blood is essential for conception and pregnancy. Other clinical manifestations of yang deficiency have been described above for Spleen yang deficiency presenting with a pale wet tongue. In this case, however, the dry tongue is also caused by Lung qi deficiency and there may be shortness of breath and a weakened voice. In severe cases there may be accumulation of fluids in the abdomen and a dry mouth and tongue resulting from fluids accumulating in the lower burner and becoming depleted in the upper burner.

PALE, BRIGHT AND SHINY

On a pale, bright and shiny tongue the coating has come off entirely and the surface of the tongue looks like freshly-plucked chicken flesh (PLATE 56). This indicates weakness of the Stomach and Spleen as well as qi and blood deficiency, all of which are of long duration. The peeling usually starts from the center of the tongue (due to Stomach deficiency) then spreads outward until it covers the entire surface. The long-standing weakness of the Stomach and Spleen will eventually induce a deficiency of qi and blood, since the Spleen is the source of blood and the Stomach is the origin of acquired qi[3] in the body.

A progressive, severe deficiency of Stomach and Spleen qi and blood deprives the tongue of nourishment and the coating gradually comes off, while no new coating is formed. The result is a tongue which is pale (due to qi and blood deficiency) and peeled bright (due to persistent weakness of the Stomach and Spleen). It should be remembered here that a peeled, red tongue indicates deficiency of the yin aspects of the body. Other clinical manifestations will be those of Spleen and Stomach deficiency, including extreme lassitude, loss of appetite and epigastric pain. In severe cases there will be emaciation and weakness of the limbs. A long-standing weakness of Stomach and Spleen will deprive the muscles of nourishment and can lead to atrophy of the muscles and extreme weakness. This type of condition is sometimes associated with neurological disorders, such as multiple sclerosis.

Red

The tongue body color described as red always indicates a pathological condition. As mentioned above, this is a color that is redder than the normal pale red of a healthy tongue. Historically, the study of red tongues was primarily an outgrowth of the development of the identification of patterns according to the four levels: the defensive qi, qi, nutritive qi and blood levels of disease. This system of identification of patterns was fully described in the early Qing dynasty (APPENDIX II). The four levels identification of patterns provides a framework for the analysis of clinical manifestations, prognosis and treatment of warm-febrile diseases. Each of the four levels represents a different degree of depth in the penetration of heat into the body, the defensive qi level being the most superficial, and the blood level being the deepest and most serious.

In all diseases from externally-contracted heat the tongue body color will be red. In fact, this color always indicates heat, whether from deficiency or excess. Examination of the tongue body color provides a reliable parameter in the evaluation of clinical signs in the four levels differentiation. Changes in that color, as well as the appearance of spots, are a useful gauge of the progress and prognosis of a disease.

The distribution of red over the surface of the tongue and its changes accurately reflect the progress of a disease. In the defensive qi level only the tip of the tongue will be red, indicating that the pathogenic heat is lodged in the superficial layers of the body. In the qi stage the tongue color is red all over. In the nutritive qi and blood stages the tongue color is dark red with red or purple spots.

In chronic, interior conditions a tongue that is entirely red always indicates heat at the nutritive qi or blood levels, although this heat need not necessarily have been derived from an attack by external heat.

Other clinical manifestations associated with a red tongue will vary considerably depending on the particular condition and where the heat is localized. The general signs of heat include redness of the face and eyes, fever, thirst, dry lips, constipation, dark urine and a rapid pulse. Clinical manifestations for different kinds of red tongues when only certain areas of the tongue are red are described below.

The internally-retained heat that is indicated by a red tongue may be excess or deficiency heat depending on whether or not the tongue has a coating. This is the first thing to establish when we see a red tongue: if it has a coating with root (whatever its color) it is due to heat from excess; if it has no coating (or a coating without root) it is due to heat from deficiency. Unless otherwise noted, the discussion of the clinical significance of other characteristics below assumes a red tongue with coating.

The specific clinical significance of a red tongue — beyond indicating the presence of heat — depends upon other signs and on the distribution of the color on the surface of the tongue, which should be interpreted with reference to tongue topography: the tip corresponding to the Heart, the sides to the Liver and Gallbladder, the center to the Stomach and Spleen, the area between the tip and center to the Lungs, and the root to the Kidneys.

RED TIP

A red tongue tip is usually associated with Heart fire; the darker the tip, the more severe the condition. If the entire tongue is red or dark red and the tip is redder still, the presence of heat in the nutritive qi or blood levels and Heart fire is indicated. This condition is usually associated with persisting emotional problems such as depression, repressed anger, or resentment. Over a long period of time these emotions cause stagnation of qi, which becomes constrained or "compressed." The compression of qi gives rise to heat, much as the increase in pressure of a gas (similar in nature to qi) leads to an increase in its temperature.

The heat is often generated in the chest, which is the seat of qi and where the Heart lies. This leads to Heart fire with symptoms of mental restlessness, irritability, insomnia, a feeling of oppression in the chest, depression and a red tongue with a redder tip (PLATES 18 & 47).

In less severe cases the tongue body color may be normal and only the tip will be red. Here, too, the Heart has fire but in a milder form caused by less intense emotional problems. In some cases the tongue body color may be normal and only the tip slightly red. This is often caused by lack of sleep and does not necessarily indicate Heart fire. A Chinese study showed that there is a high correlation between insomnia and a red tip or red points on the tip.[4] The survey found that 80.6% of people suffering from dream-disturbed sleep have either a red tip or red points on the tip, while 78.7% of those suffering from insomnia have the same sign. In the case of both insomnia and dream-disturbed sleep, the percentage rises to 85.2%. Interestingly, the study also found that fewer than 10 red points on the tip have no clinical significance.

A red tongue tip due to Heart fire must be distinguished from one due to Lung heat. If the very tip of the tongue is red, Heart fire is indicated; but if a larger area of the tip is red and the coating thin and yellow, this indicates Lung heat (PLATE 49).

RED SIDES

When the sides of the tongue are redder than the red tongue body, and also slightly swollen, Liver yang or Liver fire is indicated. This condition, like Heart fire, usually arises from long-standing emotional problems, particularly those involving anger or resentment. The patient will probably be irritable and prone to anger, present with headaches, dizziness, a bitter taste in the mouth, constipation, a wiry pulse and a red tongue with red sides (PLATES 2 & 7). This type of tongue should not be confused with another in which the sides are swollen over a larger area and the tongue body color is usually normal (PLATE 8). These latter signs indicate chronic Spleen qi or Spleen yang deficiency. This is an example of the same area of the tongue relating to two different Organs, with the conditions distinguished by different combinations of tongue signs.

RED CENTER

The central area of the tongue corresponds to the Stomach and Spleen. If the center of the tongue is red and the remainder of the tongue has a normal color, heat in the Stomach is usually indicated (PLATE 20). In this case the patient would display such symptoms as a burning sensation in the epigastrium, thirst, constipation, dry lips, swelling and pain in the gums and a rapid pulse.

If the center of the tongue is reddish-purple it indicates blood stasis in the Stomach. The presentation includes severe, stabbing pain in the epigastrium, vomiting of dark blood, bleeding gums and a firm pulse (one which is deep and hidden, but wiry and long at the deep level).

If the center is red and peeled it indicates Stomach yin deficiency leading to heat with symptoms of dry mouth, a burning sensation in the lips, thirst with a desire for warm fluids, or to drink in small sips,[5] dry stool, dry throat, epigastric pain and a rapid, fine pulse (PLATE 20). The condition of Stomach yin deficiency is commonly found in clinical practice. It arises from chronic overwork with irregular eating habits, such as eating late at night, irregular meals, and eating in a hurry or while worrying. The Stomach is the source of fluids in the body and Stomach yin deficiency implies a state of exhaustion of body fluids with related symptoms of dryness. Stomach yin deficiency often precedes Kidney yin deficiency, at which point the whole tongue becomes red and peeled, rather than just the center as in the case of Stomach yin deficiency.

RED ROOT

It is unusual for only the root to be red since a red root indicates a state of Kidney yin deficiency alone. Kidney yin is the basis of all the yin energies of the body; when Kidney yin is deficient, all the yin of the body is deficient and the whole tongue becomes red and peeled. However, there are cases when only the root is red and peeled (PLATE 43).

If the whole tongue is red and the root is redder and peeled, this indicates the presence of Kidney yin deficiency with a preponderance of pathological minister fire from deficiency within the Kidneys. The symptoms include malar flush, mental restlessness, night sweating, afternoon fever, insomnia, scanty, dark urine, dry throat at night, dry stool, excessive sexual desire, nocturnal emissions and a rapid, fine pulse.

RED AND WET

A red tongue indicates heat and will usually also be dry, since heat dries the body's fluids. However, it is not uncommon to see a red tongue that is also moist (PLATE 2). This type of tongue usually occurs when there is both heat in the nutritive qi level and retention of dampness. This often happens when there is Liver yang rising or Liver fire, making the tongue red, and deficient Spleen qi, leading to the formation of dampness. In fact, deficient Spleen qi may often be caused by rising Liver yang or Liver fire.

A red, wet tongue may also indicate deficient yang qi, with false yang "floating" upward. In this rather rare condition yang qi is extremely deficient; the yin and yang energies separate so that what little yang remains in the body floats upward, making the tongue red. At the same time, the deficient yang qi fails to transform and transport the fluids so that they accumulate on the tongue and make it wet. This is a condition of true cold (reflected in the tongue's wetness) and false heat (reflected in its redness). The tongue will also be tender, rather soft and flaccid, which is a sign of deficiency (in this case, yang deficiency).

Finally, if a red tongue is only slightly moist it simply means that the heat has not been present in the body long enough to dry up the fluids. This is a favorable indication, in contrast to the situation in which the tongue is both red and dry.

Clinical manifestations in the case of a red and wet tongue will generally be those of rising Liver yang and deficiency of Spleen qi with retention of dampness. The symptoms include headache, dizziness, a tendency to get angry quickly, red face, abdominal distension, poor digestion, a tendency toward retaining mucus in the nasal passages or chest and a slippery, wiry pulse.

RED AND DRY

If a tongue is red, dry and has a coating, excess heat in the interior is indicated. If the same tongue has no coating, it indicates deficient yin with exhaustion of the body fluids and deficiency heat.

The dryness in each of these two conditions has a different cause. With interior excess heat the dryness is due to burning of the body fluids by heat. The tongue has a yellow coating (PLATE 18). With yin deficiency the dryness is due to exhaustion of the body fluids, which are part of the yin of the body. The tongue has no coating. This latter type of tongue indicates deficiency of the Kidney yin over a long period of time; the body fluids become exhausted because the Kidneys fail to generate them (PLATE 26).

Other clinical manifestations of interior excess heat will vary widely depending on the condition and the place where the heat is localized. General signs of interior excess heat include redness of the face and eyes, usually fever, constipation, dark urine, thirst and a rapid, full pulse. The clinical manifestations of yin deficiency were previously described.

RED AND SHINY

A red tongue which looks bright and shiny like a mirror always indicates a state of yin deficiency and a lack of body fluids. This type of tongue may appear after profuse sweating in the course of an acute disease. It reflects a worsening of the condition due to the exhaustion of the yin fluids. In chronic cases it can appear in the late stages of a long-standing disease which has weakened the Stomach and Kidney fluids (PLATE 11).

If, in addition to being red and shiny, the root of the tongue is dry, it indicates deficiency of Kidney yin; if only the center of the tongue is dry, it indicates deficiency of Stomach yin.

This type of tongue can also form as a consequence of the excessive use of a drying Chinese herbal medicine. With biomedical pharmaceuticals this tongue can appear after a course of therapy with antibiotics. This is due to the fact that, from the perspective of Chinese physiology, these drugs injure the yin fluids of the Stomach and Intestines.

The clinical manifestations in a chronic condition displaying this type of tongue will be those of Stomach and/or Kidney yin deficiency. The symptoms of Stomach yin deficiency include dryness of the mouth, thirst, a burning sensation in the lips with a desire for warm liquids or to drink in small sips, dryness of the throat, loss of appetite, constipation with dry stool and a rapid, fine pulse. Stomach yin deficiency is often transmitted to the Large Intestine, in which case there is constipation with small, dry stool that is difficult to pass. This pattern is often found either in the elderly or among thin, emaciated patients. The condition is frequently encountered in clinical practice today and is due to poor and irregular eating habits, excessive consumption of spicy foods which injure Stomach yin and excessive consumption of sour foods, such as oranges, grapefruit, vinegar, yoghurt and pickles.

If the condition is one of Kidney yin deficiency as well as Stomach yin deficiency the clinical manifestations can also include tinnitus, deafness, lower back pain, vertigo, impaired memory, night sweats, nocturnal dryness in the mouth and throat, thirst, heat in the five centers (a feeling of heat in the sternum, palms of the hands and soles of the feet), nocturnal emissions, constipation, dark urine and a floating, empty and rapid pulse.

RED AND SCARLET

A red tongue with a scarlet shade, bright and tending toward pink, is usually also shiny. If it is shiny, yin deficiency is indicated. This type of tongue is most frequently associated with Lung yin or Heart yin deficiency, in which cases it could also be scarlet only in the anterior part (for the Lungs), or at the tip (for the Heart) (PLATE 26).

This type of tongue is more often found in elderly or middle-aged people. Lung yin and Heart yin deficiencies have different etiologies. Lung yin deficiency is almost always the consequence of long-standing Lung qi deficiency. Lung yin deficiency, characterized by dryness of the Lungs, is often caused by chronic overwork, a sedentary occupation which imposes a strained position on the Lungs or spending long periods of time in very hot and dry environments (such as occurs in many modern offices). It is particularly common among people such as teachers whose profession requires much talking.

Heart yin deficiency is most often caused by deep emotional problems (e.g., continuous worry, anxiety and grief, especially from difficult relationships) in conjunction with overwork or excessive physical strain, which weakens the Kidney yin. Deficiency of Kidney yin will lead to the development of deficiency heat in the Heart. In terms of the five phases, this is a situation of "water not controlling fire." In this case the very tip of the tongue may become scarlet red.

Clinical manifestations of Lung yin deficiency include a dry cough, or a cough producing scanty mucus which may be blood-tinged, dryness of the mouth and throat, night sweats, heat in the five centers and a fine, rapid pulse.

Clinical manifestations of Heart yin deficiency include mental restlessness, heat in the five centers, night sweats, insomnia, dryness of the throat, palpitations, impaired memory and a fine, rapid pulse.

RED POINTS OR SPOTS

Points and spots are distinguished by their size, the former being smaller than the latter. Each has a slightly different clinical significance, but both are indicative of the pathological state of the papillae. From the ancient Chinese perspective, the papillae are formed by arousal of the fire of the gate of vitality ascending to the surface of the tongue and causing the papillae to turn red. When there is a pathological, excess fire in the body (not the physiological fire of the gate of vitality), it rises to the tongue and causes the papillae to rise from the tongue surface forming what the ancient Chinese doctors called points *(diǎn)* or spots *(bān)*. Both points and spots are usually red, but they can also be pale red, white, purple or even black. They are usually found on a red tongue but can also be found on a pale or purple tongue.

The clinical significance of points and spots depends upon many factors such as their color, the color of the tongue body upon which they occur, and their distribution. Generally, red points indicate heat in the blood if they are raised from the tongue surface and quite pointed. Red spots indicate both heat and blood stasis; the larger the spots, the more severe is the stasis. To further clarify the clinical significance of red points and spots, several different types of tongues must be distinguished.

Red with Red Points

A red tongue with red points always indicates the presence of heat in the blood. The distribution of the points shows the location of the disease.

On the Tip — Red points on the tongue tip indicate the presence of Heart fire, usually due to emotional problems such as deep anxiety or long-standing grief (PLATE 47). The patient with this type of tongue is likely to suffer from insomnia and anxiety and have a rapid, full and overflowing pulse.

Of course, the clinical manifestations need not always be so severe, as there are different degrees of severity reflected in the number and intensity of color of the points. The deeper the color and the more numerous the points, the more serious is the condition.

On the Sides — Red points on the sides of the tongue indicate the presence of Liver fire or Liver yang rising. In this case the points are distributed as a thin line on the edges of the tongue, or on one side only. If they occur only on the right side, they indicate heat in the Gallbladder; if only on the left side, they indicate Liver fire (PLATE 4 & ILLUSTRATION 5-1a).

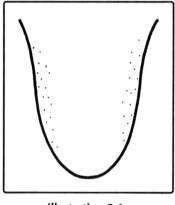 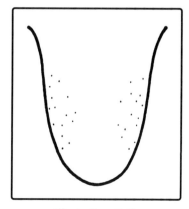

Illustration 5-1a	**Illustration 5-1b**

This condition is often due to emotional problems such as long-standing anger and resentment, and also to excessive consumption of spicy or greasy, deep-fried foods, or alcohol. Clinical manifestations include headaches, redness of the face and eyes, a bitter taste in the mouth, dizziness, tinnitus, dark urine, constipation, irritability with a tendency to quick anger and shouting, and a wiry, rapid and full pulse. If there is also heat in the Gallbladder, there will be hypochondriac pain, sighing and jaundice.

On the Sides, Central Area — Red points on the sides, but only towards the central area of the tongue, indicate heat in the Stomach and/or Spleen (ILLUSTRA-TION 5-1b). Red points in this area should be clearly distinguished from those per-taining to Liver fire (COMPARE ILLUSTRATIONS 5-1a & 5-1b).

Clinical manifestations of Stomach heat include thirst, a feeling of heat, exces-sive appetite, bleeding gums, epigastric pain, and a wiry pulse on the right middle position.

Clinical manifestations of Spleen heat include thirst, left hypochondriac pain, dry stool, dry lips, a feeling of heat and a reddish color on the forehead.

On the Root — Red points on the root may occur with or without a tongue coating. If there is a yellow coating, the presence of heat either in the Bladder or Intestines is indicated. If there is no coating, red points on the root indicate the presence of "reckless fire" (pathological minister fire) within the Kidneys arising from deficiency of Kidney yin.

Because red points on the root with a coating indicate heat in the lower burner generally, one must distinguish between heat in the Bladder or Intestines on the basis of the symptoms and the pulse. If there is heat in the Bladder the symptoms will include a burning sensation during urination, dark, scanty urine and a rapid, wiry pulse in the proximal or rear pulse position on the left wrist. This condition commonly occurs in people with the biomedical diagnosis of cystitis or urethritis.

If there is heat in the Intestines the tongue will be red, the coating yellow and there will be red points on the root, as above. The symptoms associated with this condition, however, will also include lower abdominal pain, constipation, perhaps alternating with diarrhea, blood in the stool, a burning sensation in the anus, dark urine and a rapid, full and wiry pulse in both proximal positions.

The diagnosis is more difficult in women since the lower burner also contains the Womb. From a biomedical perspective, heat in a woman's lower burner could overlap with disorders of the bladder, intestines, uterus, fallopian tubes or ovaries. A red tongue with red points on the root is in fact frequently seen in cases of inflammation of one of the pelvic organs.

Moreover, tongue diagnosis can be used to distinguish cases of true infection from those of non-infectious inflammation. Very often a patient may have symptoms of infection, which in modern biomedicine is attributed to a pathogenic organism and treated with antibiotics, while in fact the condition is caused by a combination of deficiency and stagnation of qi, giving rise to abdominal pain. In most cases of true infection the tongue will be red, the coating thick, yellow and perhaps greasy, and there will be red points on the tongue's root. If there is no infection the tongue will usually not be red, the coating not thick (although it may still be yellow), and the root of the tongue will not exhibit red points. Additionally, the pulse and other symptoms will point to the presence of deficiency.

Red with Red Spots

Spots, larger than points, can be red, dark red, purple or black. Spots indicate heat with blood stasis. Dark red or black spots indicate a greater degree of heat than red spots, while purple ones indicate a greater degree of blood stasis than do red spots. As with red points, the distribution of the spots enables the practitioner to locate the problem.

On the Tip — Red spots on the tongue tip indicate the presence of heat and blood stasis in the Heart. This is usually due to long-standing emotional problems such as anxiety and grief. Symptoms include a stabbing or pricking pain in the chest, purple lips, palpitations, sweating, coldness in the limbs, particularly the hands, and a knotted pulse.

On the Sides — Red spots on the sides of the tongue indicate the presence of heat and blood stasis in the Liver. The Liver stores the blood and when the Liver qi is constrained it may lead to stagnation of Liver qi, which, over a long period of time, will cause stasis of Liver blood. This is usually caused by emotional problems such as resentment and repressed anger.

Clinical manifestations include hypochondriac pain or lower abdominal pain which is fixed and boring or stabbing in nature. If there is any bleeding (such as menstrual, abnormal uterine or gastrointestinal tract bleeding) the blood will be purple or brown in color and perhaps contain clots. Stasis of Liver blood commonly affects the reproductive system in women causing dysmenorrhea, dark-clotted menstrual blood and severe pain. Severe and long-standing cases of stasis of Liver blood in women can lead to the formation of uterine fibroids or even cancer. In all cases of stasis of Liver blood the pulse will be wiry or firm.

On the Root — Red spots on the root indicate the presence of blood stasis in the lower burner, i.e., the Bladder, Intestines or Womb (PLATE 12).

The etiology and clinical manifestations are the same as those of red points on the root. The only difference is that with spots there will be blood stasis as well as heat. This will always involve the presence of more intense and fixed pain, which is persistent and boring or stabbing in nature.

If there is Bladder involvement the patient may complain of intense pain during urination. The urine may contain blood, and the pulse will be wiry at the proximal position of the left wrist.

If the Intestines are affected the patient may complain of stabbing lower abdominal pain, dark blood in the stool, and constipation with pain. The patient's pulse will be wiry at the proximal position on both wrists.

If the Womb is affected the patient will complain of painful periods, with pain that is stabbing and severe. The pain will be more severe before the periods and slightly relieved by their onset. Menstrual blood will be dark, with clots, and the patient will have a wiry pulse.

Red Points in Externally-Contracted Diseases

Red points acquire a particular importance in externally-contracted diseases caused by an attack of wind-heat or damp-heat. The distribution, intensity of color and number of red points on the tongue accurately reflect the intensity and location of the external pathogenic factor.

It was previously explained that the outside of the tongue corresponds to the exterior portions of the body, i.e., the skin, muscles and channels. The central surface of the tongue corresponds to the interior portions of the body, i.e., the Organs. On a vertical plane, the front part of the tongue corresponds to the top of the body (upper burner), the middle part to the middle portion (middle burner), and the root to the lower portion of the body (lower burner). In the context of externally-contracted diseases, the front part of the tongue, besides corresponding to the upper burner, also corresponds to the exterior portions of the body. For example, a thin, white and wet coating in the front part of the tongue may indicate that wind-cold is attacking the upper burner; it may also indicate that an external pathogenic factor is in the exterior layers of the body.

Red points frequently appear when there is externally-contracted heat, and they can appear on a red, a normal or even a pale tongue. This depends on the condition of the patient prior to the attack. If the patient has had a condition of blood or yang deficiency before the attack of external pathogenic heat, there will be red points on a pale tongue. However, if the pathogenic heat is not expelled but remains in the body, the tongue itself will tend to turn red.

On the Front — Red points on the front (over an area larger than the very tip) indicate an attack of external pathogenic heat in the first stage, affecting only the upper burner and the exterior energetic layers of the body (PLATE 36). In the case of externally-contracted wind-heat, it corresponds to the defensive qi level in the system of the four levels identification of patterns, and to the upper burner stage in the three burners identification of patterns (APPENDICES II & III). From a biomedical perspective, this type of tongue is frequently seen in pharyngitis, upper respiratory tract infections with fevers, and influenza. All of these conditions can be regarded as externally-contracted wind-heat, manifested on the tongue as red points on the front. This is seen with particular frequency in children, whose tongues are very prone to develop red points.

As far as prognosis is concerned, the presence of red points on the front indicate that the heat is still in the outer layers of the body and therefore fairly easy to expel. Red points extending toward the center of the tongue indicate that the externally-contracted heat has progressed inward to the interior of the body, at which stage it is more dangerous and difficult to expel.

On the Sides — Red points on the sides also indicate externally-contracted heat affecting only the exterior energetic layers of the body (PLATE 36). In the case of wind-heat, an attack of this kind corresponds to the defensive qi level of the four levels. This differs from red points on the front in that the latter indicate that the location of the wind-heat is in the upper burner where it affects the exterior energetic layers controlled by the Lungs. Red points on the sides, however, simply indicate the presence of wind-heat in the exterior energetic layers of the body, not necessarily in the upper burner. If the red points move inward toward the center of the tongue it means that the pathogenic factor has progressed more deeply inward and become an interior symptom.

On the Left or Right of the Center — Red points on the left or right side of the center (PLATE 10) indicate externally-contracted wind-heat in the intermediate stage where it is called "half-interior, half-exterior." The expression "half-interior, half-exterior" refers to the location of the disease in an intermediate stage between exterior and interior. This is also called the lesser yang pattern in the context of the six stages identification of patterns (APPENDIX I). The lesser yang pattern typically affects the Triple Burner and Gallbladder channels, with accompanying bitter taste in the mouth, dry throat, blurred vision, alternating chills and fever (a key symptom), hypochondriac pain and a wiry pulse. The tongue will present with red points either on the right or left side (typically on the right), and will exhibit a white, slippery coating on the right side alone.

This type of pattern is often observed in children who frequently suffer from ear infections or sore throats. It can also develop from the greater yang pattern of a wind-cold attack. Typically, the child may come down with a severe cold with fever and cough (greater yang pattern) and later develop an earache, alternating chills and fever, and vomiting (lesser yang pattern). Red points on one or both sides of the tongue are also frequently seen in children's diseases involving rashes, such as chicken pox and measles.

Pale Red or White Points — Pale red or white points may be found on the tongue. Pale red points are frequently seen around the central surface of the tongue. They are usually found on a normal or pale tongue and indicate the presence of very slight heat in the Stomach, but with deficient Stomach and Spleen qi.

White or very pale *concave* points do not indicate heat at all, but the presence of cold. They may also be found around the center of the tongue, indicating that the cold is present in the Stomach (PLATE 14).

RED WITH PRICKLES

The tongue is said to have "prickles" when the papillae are bigger than normal and are raised, like thorns or the stiff hairs of a brush. These are most commonly found with a red tongue (PLATE 27). In the Discussion of Warm-febrile Diseases it is said, "No matter what color the tongue body, prickles indicate heat in the upper burner."[6] Some of the papillae are said to be derived from the fire of the gate of vitality rising to meet the Lungs, which gives rise to soft white hair-like papillae in the center of the tongue. The prickles mentioned here are a pathological degeneration of the normal soft white hair-like papillae. Prickles are formed from the action of pathological heat, usually in the Lungs, which controls the formation of normal papillae. In clinical practice prickles can also indicate heat in the middle burner, particularly in the Stomach.

Prickles, then, indicate the presence of heat at the nutritive qi level, either in the upper burner (Lungs) or middle burner (Stomach). The localization and clinical manifestations associated with the prickles will vary accordingly.

Heat in the upper burner corresponds to heat in the Lungs. The prickles will be located more in the area between the tip and the center of the tongue. They could also be found all across the center of the tongue, or just around the center, as these areas may also correspond to the chest. Other clinical signs include fever, rapid breathing, a cough with yellow sputum, thirst, dryness of the throat and a rapid, full pulse. Prickles may also be found in chronic cases, such as chronic bronchitis, where there is a cough with yellow mucus, shortness of breath and a rapid, slippery pulse.

Heat in the middle burner corresponds to heat in the Stomach (PLATE 27). The prickles are located in the center of the tongue, and usually there is a wide crack in the center with yellow prickles inside it. The patient is likely to have epigastric pain, vomiting, hunger, swollen and bleeding gums, constipation, thirst and a rapid, full pulse. From a modern biomedical perspective, a patient with these symptoms is very likely to have, or to be developing, a gastric ulcer.

RED WITH A PURPLE SPOT IN THE CENTER

A red tongue with a purple spot in its central surface indicates the presence of heat with blood stasis in the Stomach. This condition is caused by poor dietary habits such as eating in a hurry, worrying while eating or going back to work immediately after eating. This condition is often associated with a great amount of stress and worry.

Clinical manifestations include pain and distension of the epigastrium, pain of a fixed and boring nature, vomiting of dark brown blood, pain that becomes worse when pressure is applied, acid regurgitation, constipation and a full, tight pulse.

RED AND PEELED

A red, peeled tongue has no coating at all. It looks like freshly-plucked chicken flesh. When the Stomach qi is weak the coating is not formed and, in time, comes off entirely (PLATES 3, 13, 48 & 59). When the entire tongue is peeled, it indicates that the long-standing deficiency involves Kidney yin as well, with the presence of heat from yin deficiency.

The relationship between the Stomach yin and Kidney yin is one of mutual assistance. The Stomach is the source of all the body fluids, while the Kidneys control the transformation of the body fluids. The yin fluids of the Stomach and Kidneys therefore have the same source, and a persistent deficiency of Stomach yin will eventually cause a deficiency of Kidney yin. Kidney yin deficiency may be regarded as a later and more serious stage of Stomach yin deficiency. These conditions result from poor dietary habits (such as irregular eating, eating late at night and excessive consumption of sour foods) and from a life of overwork, stress and anxiety. Stomach yin deficiency is manifested in an absence of coating, and Kidney yin deficiency in a red body color. Other clinical signs vary depending upon the predominant condition.

Dark Red

The clinical significance of the dark red (also called deep red) tongue is the same as that of the red tongue; the darker color simply indicates a more serious and advanced stage of heat. The darker the shade of red, the more heat there is. Thus, whatever has been said above about the various types of red tongues applies as well to dark red tongues.

A survey of 300 cases of dark red tongue bodies in China showed that they are correlated with diseases of the digestive tract in people over 40 years of age. Experiments also revealed that the microcirculation of dark red tongues is better than that of purple tongues, but worse than that of red tongues.[7] This correlates exactly with the traditional Chinese view which places the dark red tongue body color between the red and reddish-purple color in terms of seriousness of the underlying condition.

DARK RED AND DRY IN THE CENTER

A dark red tongue with a dry central surface and a coating indicates heat from excess in the nutritive qi or blood levels. This condition is specifically localized in the Stomach when there is Stomach fire. The dryness results from the fire having burned up the body fluids. This condition can be caused by excessive consumption of hot and spicy foods, or greasy, fried foods. It can also result from excessive consumption of alcohol.

A dark red tongue with a dry central surface and no coating indicates heat arising from deficiency of Kidney and Stomach yin. The dryness results from exhaustion of the body's fluids.

Note that different causes in these two cases both result in dryness. When there is heat from excess, the dryness is due to the burning of the body fluids by heat. When there is deficiency heat, the dryness arises from exhaustion of the yin fluids from the general deficiency of Stomach and Kidney yin. The cause of a dark red, dry, and peeled tongue is nearly always overwork in the sense of working long hours without adequate rest and with irregular eating habits.

Clinical manifestations when there is a coating include epigastric pain, bleeding gums, a burning sensation in the epigastrium, restlessness, thirst, constipation and a full, overflowing and rapid pulse. Clinical signs when there is no coating include thirst, dryness of the mouth at night, lower back pain, tinnitus, heat in the five centers, night sweats, afternoon feverishness, malar flush and a pulse that is rapid and fine, or floating and empty.

Purple

A purple tongue body always indicates blood stasis. A tongue turns purple only after a rather long period of time and indicates that the pathological process is of long duration. There are two basic types of purple tongues: the bluish purple and the reddish purple. The former derives from a pale tongue and the latter from a red or dark red one (ILLUSTRATION 5-2).

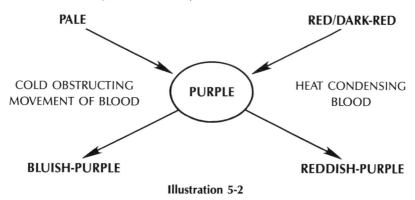

Illustration 5-2

The clinical significance of a bluish purple and reddish purple tongue is the same as that of a pale and red tongue respectively, except that they also indicate the presence of blood stasis, the cause of which is different for each tongue shade. With a bluish purple tongue, the stasis is due to obstruction from internal cold; with a reddish purple tongue, it is due to heat in the blood, which causes the blood to coagulate and stagnate. Within these two basic types of purple tongues, several variations should be noted.

REDDISH PURPLE

A reddish purple tongue is usually dry. It indicates extreme heat in the nutritive qi and blood levels, with blood stasis and consumption of body fluids (PLATES 21, 27, 48 & 59).

If the whole tongue is purple, there is extreme heat in the Organs.[8]

If the tongue is purple, dry and cracked, it indicates extreme heat, which is difficult to treat.[9]

The long-standing retention of heat in the body injures the qi and body fluids. As a result of the fluids' exhaustion, the blood loses nourishment and moisture. Similarly, the qi cannot perform its function of moving the blood. The result is blood stasis and a purple coloration of the tongue body. The exhaustion of the body fluids also dries and sometimes cracks the tongue.

Clinical manifestations vary greatly depending on the predominant pathology. The general signs and symptoms of blood stasis include fixed pain that is stabbing or boring in nature, menstrual bleeding with dark purple and clotted blood, aggravation of the pain at night and a wiry, firm or choppy pulse. In addition to these general symptoms there will be some signs of heat, which vary according to its location in the body.

Reddish Purple Tip

A reddish purple tongue tip indicates blood stasis in the Heart with heat. This is a serious condition which usually occurs over a long period of time. From a biomedical perspective, it is often associated with angina pectoris and coronary heart disease. The primary clinical manifestations of heat and blood stasis in the Heart include pain in the chest of a pricking or stabbing nature, which may extend to the back or along the medial aspect of the left arm to the little finger, chest congestion, palpitations, purple lips, a flushed face, a desire to open windows for fresh air and a knotted, firm or choppy pulse, possibly overflowing in the left distal position. The tongue will also have red or purple spots on the tip indicating blood stasis in the Heart.

Reddish Purple Sides

A reddish color with purple or red spots on the sides of the tongue indicates heat and blood stasis of the Liver. This is usually a consequence of stagnation of Liver qi over a long period of time, and is a rather common pathological condition. Liver qi and blood are very prone to stagnation, particularly in women.

The clinical manifestations of this condition include hypochondriac pain, headaches of a stabbing nature in the temples and eyes, dizziness, tinnitus, a bitter taste in the mouth and lower abdominal pain of a twisting or boring nature, and of fixed location. In women other manifestations include dysmenorrhea, pain and distension of the breasts before the onset of periods, premenstrual tension, irregular menstruation with dark purple and clotted blood, and a wiry pulse.

The most common causes of this condition are anger over a long period of time and frustration and repressed feelings, combined with excessive consumption of spicy and/or greasy foods and/or alcohol.

DARK REDDISH PURPLE

Generally, the clinical significance of this type of tongue is the same as that of the reddish purple tongue, except that its darker color indicates extreme heat with blood stasis (PLATE 13). This type of tongue has two variants: dry and wet.

Dark Reddish Purple and Dry

A dark reddish purple tongue that is dry indicates heat in the blood and blood stasis. The clinical signs are the same as those for the reddish purple tongue described above, and depend on the localization of the heat and stasis, i.e., in the Heart or in the Liver.

Dark Reddish Purple and Wet

A dark reddish purple tongue that is wet indicates heat in the nutritive qi level and blood stasis. This type of tongue differs from the dry one in the depth of the heat: heat in the nutritive qi level is a more superficial level of penetration than is heat in the blood. This is because blood and the body fluids have the same origin and heat in the blood level will tend to burn the body fluids, resulting in dryness of the tongue. If the heat is only in the nutritive qi level, the body fluids are not yet necessarily affected and the tongue is therefore wet. There will still be blood stasis because of the failure of nutritive qi to move the blood.

With the exception of this difference, the clinical manifestations for both dry and wet tongues will be similar. These manifestations have been described above for the reddish purple tongue.

REDDISH PURPLE AND DISTENDED

A reddish purple distended tongue (PLATE 21) usually indicates heat and blood stasis, commonly in the Liver and/or Heart, caused by excessive consumption of alcohol over a long period of time. The tongue is usually redder on the sides and tip. The tongue is distended because of the extreme heat in the Heart. Because the tongue is an offshoot of the Heart, extreme heat in that Organ can cause the tongue to swell. (It may also do so from completely different causes; see chapter 6.)

Clinical manifestations are those of heat in the Liver and Heart with blood stasis, previously described. There will also be symptoms of intense heat (since alcohol is very hot), such as a very red face (or a reddish purple one indicating blood stasis in addition to heat), thirst, constipation, dark urine and a rapid, over-flowing pulse.

BLUISH PURPLE

A bluish purple tongue (PLATES 14 & 22) evolves from a pale tongue over a very long period of time. It indicates internal cold with blood stasis. Internal cold is an obstructive force, preventing the smooth flow of blood. A bluish purple tongue, like a pale tongue, can be caused by excessive consumption of cold and raw foods and chronic exposure to cold and damp environments occurring against a background of yang deficiency.

Clinical manifestations accompanying a bluish purple tongue are generally associated with long-standing deficiency of yang with internal cold and blood stasis. These manifestations include chilliness, coldness of the limbs, a bluish tint to the lips, abdominal pain, loose stool, clear and copious urine, sweating, impotence in men, dysmenorrhea in women, and a deep, firm, slow or choppy pulse. Other clinical signs vary depending on the localization of the internal cold.

Bluish Purple Tip

A bluish purple tongue tip, indicating cold and blood stasis in the Heart, is due to long-standing deficiency of Heart yang. Such deficiency leads to internal cold in the chest and consequent blood stasis there as a result of the failure of Heart yang to move the blood.

Clinical manifestations include chills, cold hands, a bluish purple tint to the lips, stabbing pain in the chest extending to the back or along the medial aspect of the left arm to the little finger, spontaneous sweating, palpitations and a knotted, deep pulse.

Bluish Purple Central Surface

A bluish purple central tongue surface, indicating cold and blood stasis in the Spleen, is due to chronic deficiency of Spleen yang in moving the blood.

Clinical signs include chills, a bluish tint to the lips, coldness in the limbs, abdominal pain, watery stool, loss of appetite and a slow, deep pulse.

Bluish Purple Sides in Central Area

A bluish purple color on the sides in the central area indicates stasis of blood in the chest, which can affect the Heart and/or Lungs (ILLUSTRATION 5-3). This usually occurs against a background of Heart yang deficiency.

Clinical manifestations include cyanosis of lips, stabbing pain in the chest, mental depression and anxiety, a feeling of constriction in the chest, chilliness and a choppy pulse.

Bluish Purple Root

A bluish purple tongue root, indicating cold and blood stasis in the lower burner, is due to long-standing deficiency of Kidney yang, which is often a more serious development of Spleen yang deficiency. This deficiency leads to the formation of internal cold, which obstructs the movement of blood and leads to its stasis.

Clinical manifestations include chills, coldness in the limbs, edema, impotence, watery stool, clear and copious urine, abdominal pain or lower back pain, and a deep, firm, slow pulse. Additional symptoms in women include dysmenorrhea with intense stabbing pain (due to cold in the lower burner and blood stasis), infertility, and delayed menstruation, with clotted menstrual blood.

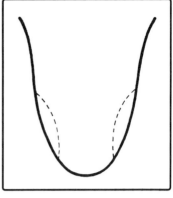

Illustration 5-3

Bluish Purple and Moist

A bluish purple tongue that is very moist, and almost dripping in severe cases, indicates internal cold from deficiency of yang leading to blood stasis. Specifically, it indicates internal cold in the Liver and Kidneys leading to stiffening of the sinews and bones, controlled respectively by the Liver and Kidneys.

Clinical manifestations reflect the pathology of internal cold in the Liver and Kidneys affecting the sinews, bones and locomotor system generally. Symptoms include chills, purple discoloration, pain and coldness in the limbs, atrophy of the musculature of the limbs, impairment of movement and even paralysis, and a deep, firm pulse. This condition corresponds to a type of atrophy disorder *(wĕi)* in Chinese medicine characterized by atrophy of the muscles and impairment of movement or paralysis.

Blue

A blue tongue indicates cold congealed internally from extreme deficiency of yang, with blood stasis. The causes of this condition are the same as those that cause a pale tongue: excessive consumption of cold and raw foods, or exposure to cold and damp weather over a long period of time occurring against a background of yang deficiency.

Clinical manifestations include chills, coldness in the limbs, watery stool, clear and copious urine and lower back pain. Additional symptoms in men include impotence, and in women dysmenorrhea with delayed periods and scanty, clotted menstrual blood.

BLUE WITHOUT COATING

A blue tongue without coating is always a sign of danger. The blue body color indicates cold congealed inside with blood stasis, and the absence of coating indicates the total collapse of qi and blood. This is one of the rare cases in which the absence of coating is due to extreme deficiency of yang rather than yin.

The clinical manifestations can vary widely and it is difficult to generalize about them. Common signs and symptoms include chills, pain and coldness in the limbs, oily sweat, lower back pain, abdominal pain, watery stool, clear and copious urine, impaired movement of limbs or even paralysis, extreme lassitude and a deep, slow, fine or scattered pulse. Other symptom in men include impotence, and in women dysmenorrhea with delayed periods and scanty, clotted menstrual blood.

BLUE CENTRAL SURFACE, SLIPPERY AND GREASY

A blue color evident only on the central surface of the tongue indicates the presence of cold internally, specifically in the Stomach and Spleen, resulting from extreme deficiency of Stomach and Spleen yang. The deficiency of Spleen yang in this case also gives rise to the formation of damp-phlegm retained in the chest.

Clinical symptoms include a feeling of constriction in the chest, abdominal distension, a cough with abundant, thick white sputum, loss of appetite, lassitude, loose stool, coldness in the limbs, nausea and vomiting, a generalized feeling of heaviness and a deep, fine, slow pulse.

BLUE TONGUE DURING PREGNANCY

A blue tongue color during pregnancy may indicate the imminent danger of miscarriage. This was noted as far back as the 7th century by Chao Yuan-Fang in *Discussion of the Origin and Symptoms of Disease*.[10] Chao observed that a blue tongue color and a red face in a pregnant woman indicate the imminent death of the fetus and survival of the mother, while a red tongue color and a blue face indicate the death of the mother and survival of the baby.

When a blue tongue is observed in a pregnant woman she should be given herbal medicine or acupuncture to tonify and warm the qi and blood even in the absence of other symptoms.

White Vesicles

Small white vesicles, usually found either in the front or center of the tongue, indicate the presence of dampness. They are like red points insofar as they are raised from the tongue surface, but are white in color (PLATE 54).

UNDERSIDE OF THE TONGUE

Examination of the underside of the tongue, and in particular the two veins under the tongue on either side of the frenulum, should be a regular part of the tongue diagnosis routine. The clinical significance of signs on this part of the tongue often augments the information gathered from examination of the tongue surface.

Method of Examination

As in the examination of the tongue surface, it is important that the tongue not be protruded with too much force, as this can cause the two veins to become distended very quickly.

Protruding the tongue to show the underside is not exactly easy, and may confound patients. The best way to proceed is to ask the patient to curl the tongue upward and gently rest its tip on the palate. Demonstration is often helpful. Examination focuses on the two veins on either side of the frenulum. One should observe their size and color (PLATE 40).

Clinical Significance

If the veins are distended but not dark, stagnation of qi is indicated. If they are dark, it indicates blood stasis; the darker the color, the more severe the stasis. Although the condition could be in any part of the body, these two veins most often reflect blood stasis in the upper burner, i.e., either in the Heart or the Lungs. When only one vein is distended, it signifies that the blood stasis is primarily on one side of the body (PLATE 39).

It is important to note that the veins can have a dark color indicating blood stasis even though the tongue body itself may not be dark red or purple. If the veins on the underside are dark and the remainder of the tongue body is not dark or purple, this indicates that the blood stasis is of short duration, not very severe, and primarily involves the upper burner. Examination of the veins under the tongue can therefore provide an early indication of qi or blood disorders before they effect a change in the tongue body itself.

The size of the veins should also be noted: distended veins usually indicate a condition of excess, thin ones a condition of deficiency.

Reddish purple and shiny veins indicate damp-heat at the nutritive qi level. Yellowish veins indicate turbid dampness steaming upwards (PLATE 55). White and slippery veins indicate the presence of damp-cold and are frequently seen in painful obstruction disorders.

SUMMARY

To summarize, the tongue body color is probably the single most important aspect of tongue diagnosis: it provides an immediate and clear picture of the pathological condition. Whenever there is any doubt in a diagnosis due to conflicting findings, the body color will almost always give an indication of the true condition.

- If the body is pale, it indicates a deficiency of yang or blood, depending on whether it is also slightly wet or dry.

- If the body is red, it indicates the presence of heat. This will be excess heat if there is a coating, or deficiency heat if there is no coating. Red points or spots indicate heat and blood stasis.

- If the body is purple, it indicates blood stasis, which could be from internal cold if it is bluish purple, or from heat if it is reddish purple.

- If the body is blue, it indicates blood stasis due to internal cold.

NOTES

1. Cao Bing-Zhang, *A Guide to Tongue Differentiation (Bian She zhi nan)* (1920). Reference provided by Su Xin-Ming.

2. Fu Song-Yuan, *A Collection of Tongues and Coatings.* Cited in Beijing College of Traditional Chinese Medicine, *Tongue Diagnosis in Chinese Medicine (Zhong yi she zhen)* (Beijing: People's Medical Publishing House, 1976), p. 17.

3. While the term blood in Chinese medicine refers, as does the English word blood, to a bodily fluid, it also has a much broader significance. In Chinese medicine, blood is made from the essence of food which is extracted by the Spleen. The process that culminates in the making of blood occurs in the chest under the action of the Lungs and Heart. The function of blood is to nourish and moisten. The movement of blood is dependent on the pushing action of qi, and qi in turn is dependent on the nourishing action of blood. This relationship is expressed in the maxim, "Qi is the commander of blood, and blood is the mother of qi." Therefore, if qi stagnates for a given period of time, blood stasis will result. In addition, blood also has a relation of mutual exchange and transformation with body fluids. This is because both are derived from food and drink and are considered yin. Due to this interchange between blood and fluids, and because they have the same origin, bleeding and sweating are considered to be mutually exclusive therapeutic modalities. As chapter 18 of *Spiritual Axis* observes, "[For] much bleeding, do not sweat; [for] much sweating, do not bleed." The condition of deficient blood in Chinese medicine is not equivalent to any particular disorder in modern biomedicine. Anemic conditions will in most cases be described as deficient blood in Chinese medicine, but one can have deficient blood without anemia. Deficiency of blood is common in women and can be due to insufficient consumption of "blood-strengthening" foods, overwork or hereditary weakness. Particularly in women, deficient blood has a very extensive meaning that embraces what would be called hormonal problems in modern biomedicine.

4. Qi Ying-Jie, "Observation of the Tongue in Insomnia." *Journal of Traditional Chinese Medicine (Zhong yi za zhi)* 28, no.3 (1987): 68.

5. Su Xin-Ming, personal communication.

6. Ye Tian-Shi, *Discussion of Warm-febrile Diseases.* Cited in *Tongue Diagnosis in Chinese Medicine*, p. 25.

7. Jia Yu-Hua, "Clinical and Experimental Research into the Dark Red Tongue." *Journal of Traditional Chinese Medicine (Zhong yi za zhi)* 33, no. 5 (1992): 46.

8. Liang Te-Yan, *Differentiation of Syndromes by Examination of the Tongue.* Cited in *Tongue Diagnosis in Chinese Medicine*, p. 26.

9. *A Collection of Tongues and Coatings.* Cited in *Tongue Diagnosis in Chinese Medicine*, p. 26.

10. See chapter 1, note 29.

TABLE OF TONGUE BODY COLOR

BODY COLOR	CLINICAL SIGNIFICANCE
Pale	Slightly dry: blood deficiency Wet: yang deficiency
Pale, bright and shiny	Qi and blood deficiency, particularly of Stomach and Spleen
Red	With coating: heat in the nutritive or blood levels Without coating: yin deficiency with heat
Red and wet	Heat with retention of dampness
Red and dry	With coating: heat from excess burning body fluids Without coating: deficiency heat and exhaustion of body fluids
Red and shiny	Stomach and/or Kidney yin deficiency
Red and scarlet	Lung or Heart yin deficiency
Red with red points or spots	Heat with blood stasis
Red with prickles	Heat in the nutritive level or in the upper or middle burner
Red with a purple spot in center	Blood stasis and heat in Stomach
Red and peeled	Heat from Stomach and Kidney yin deficiency
Dark red with a dry center	Stomach fire blazing or Stomach yin deficiency with heat
Reddish purple	Heat and blood stasis
Reddish purple and distended	Extreme heat with blood stasis and toxin from alcohol injuring the Heart
Bluish purple	Blood stasis from internal cold
Bluish purple and moist	Blood stasis from internal cold stiffening the tendons and bones
Blue	Severe internal cold with blood stasis
Blue without coating	Severe internal cold with stasis and exhaustion of blood
Blue central surface	Spleen yang deficiency with retention of phlegm in chest
Blue in a pregnant woman	Danger of imminent miscarriage
Distended veins on underside of tongue	Deficiency and stagnation of qi If veins also dark: blood stasis

6
Tongue Body Shape

After examination of tongue body color, examination of tongue body shape is the next most important aspect of tongue diagnosis. By shape here is meant not only the physical contours of the tongue, but also its consistency, texture and mobility.

The normal tongue body shape is neither too thin nor too swollen, and is soft and supple without being flabby. Its form tapers off toward the tip. Its surface is unbroken by cracks. The normal tongue can be extended easily and neither trembles nor quivers uncontrollably, nor is it involuntarily stiff or immobile.

From the perspective of the eight principles identification of patterns, the clinical significance of the tongue body is that it reflects deficiency or excess in the body. In addition, it reflects the state of the Organs, qi and especially the blood. The body shape may also suggest the presence of certain pathogenic factors such as dampness, phlegm or wind.

Nevertheless, the clinical significance of most tongue shapes still depends on the tongue body color. The color remains the single most revealing element and the one firm point of tongue diagnosis. In order to interpret the significance of a particular tongue body shape, reference must be made to the tongue body color. For example, a thin tongue body indicates deficiency of blood if the tongue body is pale, but deficiency of yin if it is red.

If reference must always be made to the color of the tongue body, why observe the shape of the tongue body at all? First, because it provides further information than can be gleaned from the color of the tongue body alone. And second, because a change in the tongue body shape indicates a more severe condition than if the shape were unchanged. For example, a red and peeled tongue indicates yin deficiency; but if it is also thin, this denotes a more severe condition and therefore a worse prognosis. Furthermore, in some cases the color of the tongue body will be normal while its shape is grossly abnormal; in such cases the shape of the tongue body becomes a more important factor in reaching a correct diagnosis (PLATE 8).

The following tongue body shapes will be discussed in this chapter: thin, swollen, partially swollen, stiff, flaccid, long, short, cracked, loose, deviated, numb, moving, quivering, rolled, tooth-marked, ulcerated and sore-covered.

THIN

By a thin tongue is meant one which is thinner than normal and appears shrunken (PLATES 7 & 17). The consistency of the tongue body derives from a normal supply of body fluids to the tongue. The fluids give it body. A thin tongue body therefore always suggests a deficiency of the yin substances, either blood or fluids. Sometimes the tongue can be so thin as to actually be shrunken, leaving longitudinal ridges on its surface.

The clinical significance of a thin tongue depends on the color of the tongue itself. If a tongue is both pale and thin, blood deficiency is indicated. A thin tongue that is also red indicates yin deficiency. The general clinical manifestations of blood deficiency and yin deficiency were described in chapter 5; the specific signs and symptoms will depend on the particular condition and Organ involved.

SWOLLEN

A swollen tongue is distended and larger than normal. In severe cases it can fill the whole mouth. The normal thickness and body of the tongue reflect a normal supply of blood and fluids. If the tongue is swollen, it means that too much fluid reaches it. This can occur for two different reasons: either the yang qi is deficient and fails to transform and transport the fluids, which accumulate in the tongue; or there is heat in the body, which pushes the fluids up to the tongue. The former is a passive process whereby fluids stagnate; the latter is more of an active process.

The swollen tongue is far more common than the thin one. This is because Spleen qi deficiency is an extremely common pattern, almost always leading to some degree of dampness or phlegm, which causes the tongue to swell. Even when Spleen qi deficiency leads to blood deficiency (as the Spleen and Stomach are the origin of blood), the tongue does not become thin (as you would expect from blood deficiency) because the presence of dampness or phlegm causes it to swell (ILLUSTRATION 6-1).

The clinical significance of five types of swollen tongues are recognized: pale and wet, normal color, fresh-looking red, purple and dark bluish purple.

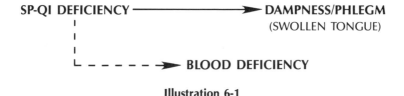

Illustration 6-1

Pale and Wet

If the body color is pale and the tongue is wet, a swollen tongue indicates deficiency of yang (specifically Spleen and Kidney yang), leading to retention of dampness (PLATE 9). This is probably the most common type of swollen tongue. When Spleen yang and/or Kidney yang are deficient, the fluids are not transformed and transported properly and therefore accumulate in the body, causing the tongue to swell. The clinical manifestations of Spleen and Kidney yang deficiencies were previously described.

A particular (and worse) type of swollen-pale-wet tongue is the one that is swollen and pale and with a sticky coating all over. This indicates the retention of dampness and/or phlegm, usually occurring against a background of Spleen deficiency. In a few cases, if the tongue is very swollen and somewhat flabby, it may indicate obstruction of the spirit by phlegm (PLATES 44 & 45).

Normal Color

If the tongue body color is normal, a swollen tongue indicates the retention of damp-heat in the Stomach and Spleen. This is also due to deficiency of Spleen qi failing to transform and transport the fluids, but in this case there is also heat. Clinical manifestations include abdominal fullness and distension, loss of appetite, a feeling of heaviness, dryness of the mouth, thirst with inability to drink very much, nausea and vomiting, abdominal pain, loose and particularly malodorous stool, a burning sensation in the anus, scanty and yellow urine, fever, headache, a rapid, fine and slippery pulse and a yellow, slippery tongue coating. (In this case the tongue coating is yellow because of the heat, and slippery because of the dampness.)

Fresh-looking Red

If the tongue body color is a fresh-looking red, a swollen tongue indicates heat in the Stomach and Heart. In this case it is Stomach heat which is transmitted to the Heart and causes the tongue to swell. (The tongue is regarded as an offshoot of the Heart.) In severe cases, there is coma due to attack upon the Pericardium by heat, with Heart fire blazing upward and clouding the consciousness. This condition is found in acute cases of febrile diseases such as meningitis. In other cases of simple Stomach and Heart heat, the clinical manifestations include thirst, a desire for cold drinks, vomiting, palpitations, insomnia, redness of the face, dry throat and a rapid, overflowing pulse.

Purple

If the tongue body color is purple, a swollen tongue indicates alcoholism with retention of damp-heat. This is called the "alcoholic toxin within" (PLATE 27).

Dark Bluish Purple

If the tongue body color is dark bluish purple, a swollen tongue indicates poisoning that is causing blood stasis.

PARTIALLY SWOLLEN

There are several types of partially swollen tongues. All are commonly found in clinical practice and an understanding of each of them will greatly aid in diagnosis.

One must first distinguish between conditions of excess and deficiency. Although both involve swelling, the mechanism underlying each is different. In conditions of deficiency the swelling is due to a deficiency of qi, which in turn causes fluids to accumulate. In conditions of excess, the swelling is due to an excess of qi or stagnant qi, which accumulates in the tongue. The main criterion for differentiating deficiency from excess swelling is the color of the tongue body: if the body is pale, the swelling is from deficiency, and if the body is red or purple, the swelling is from excess.

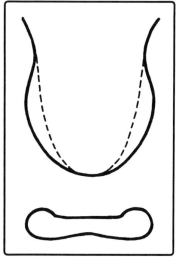

Illustration 6-2

There are several varieties of partially swollen tongues.

Swollen Edges

A tongue which is swollen on the edges, with swelling that is large and fat and more concentrated in the middle section of the tongue, is generally a tongue of pale or normal color (PLATE 8 & ILLUSTRATION 6-2).

The swelling indicates a deficiency of Spleen qi or Spleen yang. If it derives from a deficiency of Spleen yang, the edges will also be wet. This type of tongue is commonly seen in clinical practice.

The clinical manifestations of Spleen qi deficiency were previously described.

Swollen Sides

A tongue with swollen sides is usually red or purple. This type of swelling is found in a thin strip along the entire length of both sides of the tongue. This tongue differs from that with swollen edges in that the swelling is more evenly distributed along the length of the tongue body, and extends less deeply into the central tongue surface (PLATES 2, 7, 12, 23 & ILLUSTRATION 6-3).

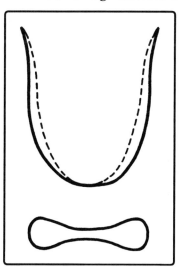

Illustration 6-3

This type of swelling indicates rising Liver yang or Liver fire. In these cases the tongue body will clearly be red, dark red or purple (if there is also blood stasis).

Other clinical signs and symptoms include dizziness, headache, blurred visioin, irritability, dryness of the mouth, a bitter taste in the mouth, constipation, dark yellow urine, and wiry pulse.

Swollen Tip

When the tongue body has a normal shape with swelling only at the very tip, a problem of the Heart is indicated. The precise clinical significance depends upon other aspects of the tongue, particularly the body color. If the tongue body color is red or dark red, a swollen tip indicates blazing Heart fire. In this case, the tip is usually also redder than the remainder of the tongue. If the body color is normal and the tip is swollen, it indicates a deficiency of Heart qi (PLATES 18 & 21).

The clinical manifestations of blazing Heart fire include thirst, a bitter taste in the mouth, insomnia, irritability, a feeling of being overly warm, redness of the face, mouth or lip ulcers and an overflowing, rapid pulse.

The clinical manifestations of Heart qi deficiency include palpitations, shortness of breath after exertion, a pale complexion and a weak or empty pulse.

Swollen Between Tip and Central Surface

A tongue with swelling in the area between the tip and the central surface (corresponding to the Lungs) will either have a normal body with swelling only in the Lung area, or a swollen tongue body with greater swelling in the Lung area (PLATES 7 & 12). This body shape is almost always found in tongues with pale or normal color.

Swelling of this kind indicates a deficiency of Lung qi with retention of damp-phlegm in the Lungs. It is commonly found in chronic conditions of Lung qi and Spleen qi deficiency, which lead to the formation and accumulation of phlegm in the Lungs.

Clinical signs and symptoms include a feeling of constriction in the chest (i.e., a feeling of suffocation or an uncomfortable feeling in the chest that the patient will find difficult to describe), perhaps a cough with abundant white sputum, poor appetite, shortness of breath, lethargy and a pulse that is empty or slightly slippery, or fine and slippery.

Swollen Along a Central Crack

The tongue body may have a crack in its center extending to the tip, on either side of which there is swelling (PLATE 8 & ILLUS-TRATION 6-4).

This type of swelling can be found on a tongue of red or normal color. On a red tongue it indicates the presence of Heart fire, and on a normal tongue it indicates Heart qi deficiency. In both cases, it indicates that

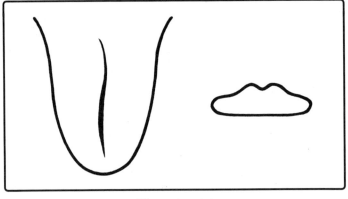

Illustration 6-4

the heart is dilated, usually due to severe overwork and constantly pushing oneself.

Clinical manifestations will be those of Heart fire or Heart qi deficiency. In addition, the patient will have marked shortness of breath, a sense of constriction in the chest and an overflowing Heart pulse.

Swollen on Half of the Tongue

When only one longitudinal half of the tongue body is swollen such that its midline does not fall in the actual center of the tongue (PLATE 16 & ILLUSTRATION 6-5), a deficiency of qi and blood in the channels of that side of the body is usually indicated. This is not related to the internal Organs, but to the channels and muscles only. Weakness of the channels on one side of the body alone is either due to progressive malnourishment of the channels from Stom-

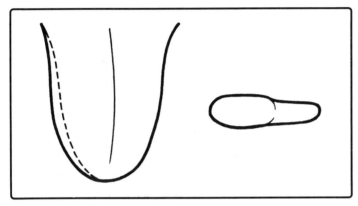

Illustration 6-5

ach and Spleen deficiency, or to injury of the channels after a prolonged febrile disease. In both cases, it is like a mild form of atrophy disorder, affecting only the channels.

Other clinical manifestations of this condition include a feeling of weakness on one side of the body (which could involve slight weakness of a leg or of the strength of grip in one hand), and a feeling of "pins and needles" or numbness on one side of the body. The needling sensation is difficult to obtain on the same side as the swelling of the tongue.

Weakness of the channels may be treated by tonifying the yang brightness channels and the Spleen, thereby tonifying the qi and blood of the channels.

Highly Localized Swelling on One Side

A tongue body that has a partial swelling in a specific area on one side should not be confused with the previously described tongue type, with swelling on one half of the tongue body (ILLUSTRATION 6-6).

Highly localized swelling on one side of the tongue indicates either a deficiency or stagnation

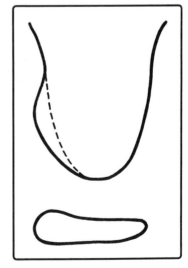

Illustration 6-6

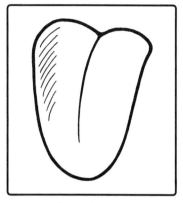

Illustration 6-7

of qi in the part of the body corresponding to the swollen area. The tongue body color is significant: if the color is normal, the swelling reflects deficiency of qi; if it is red, it reflects stagnation of qi.

The most common place where such localized swelling occurs is in the front third of one side of the tongue, in the area corresponding to the chest. This swelling is most commonly found on a tongue with pale or normal color, indicating deficiency of qi in the chest, with probable retention of dampness.

If the tongue body is red, the partial swelling indicates stagnation of qi and/or blood in the corresponding part of the human body. If the swelling is on the front third of one side, it would indicate stagnation of qi in the chest, usually resulting from emotional problems such as repressed grief or depression.

Another clinical sign common to both qi deficiency in the chest and stagnation of qi is shortness of breath and a sense of constriction in the chest. Additional signs of stagnation of qi are palpitations, depression and a wiry pulse.

Swollen on Half of Tongue Surface

When the tongue body is swollen on one longitudinal half of its upper surface, so that one half of the surface bulges upward more than the other (PLATE 32 & ILLUSTRATION 6-7), deficiency of qi in the Lung of the corresponding side is indicated. Lung deficiency can cause this type of swelling because the Lung is a bilateral Organ which can be more deficient on one side than on the other.

Clinical manifestations of Lung qi deficiency were previously described.

Hammer-shaped

A grossly misshapen tongue body, of regular size toward the root but greatly swollen in its front third like a hammer, is always an indication of a serious condition, and is often indicative of mental illness (ILLUSTRATION 6-8).

Swelling of this kind only arises after many years of pathological change. It usually reflects a serious deficiency of Spleen and Stomach qi. The causes of this condition are overwork, irregular eating, and going back to work soon after eating, and excessive sexual activity over many years.

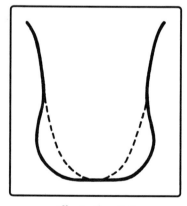

Illustration 6-8

Other clinical signs vary greatly. In any case, this type of tongue body always reflects a serious deterioration of the body's nutrient substances and energies. The condition is difficult to treat.

Swollen in Front Part

Swelling of this type occupies the whole front part of the tongue, covering approximately one-third of the body from the tip (PLATE 50). This always indicates chronic retention of phlegm in the Lungs and is frequently seen in late-onset asthma. The primary clinical manifestations include a feeling of oppression and heaviness of the chest, possible wheezing, slight breathlessness, productive cough and a slippery pulse.

STIFF

A stiff tongue has lost its suppleness and flexibility. It looks hard, and cannot move freely. This type of tongue can occur in a variety of situations. In the course of an acute disease with signs of intense heat, manifesting in high fever and delirium, a stiff tongue indicates the invasion of the Pericardium by heat. Delirium and slurred speech or aphasia may appear because the Heart is the "residence of the spirit" and controls the tongue muscle. In this case the tongue body is red or dark red.

In the course of a chronic condition, with a dry and red or dark red tongue, a stiff tongue body indicates that intense heat has injured the body fluids and led to malnourishment of sinews, muscles and channels (PLATE 27). In this situation there might also be impaired movement and stiffness of muscles. If the tongue body is red — with a redder tip — and dry, a stiff tongue body indicates blazing Heart fire, which causes the tongue fluids to dry up (PLATE 11). The *Guide to Tongue Differentiation* observes, "If the tongue is red and stiff, the Organs have extreme heat from excess."[1]

If a stiff tongue is not red but pale or of normal color, it indicates the presence of internal wind. This is frequently seen in patients who have suffered an attack of wind-stroke (a diagnosis which often overlaps with that of cerebral vascular accident in modern biomedicine) and have hemiplegia with or without asymmetry of the face. Wind-stroke, from the perspective of Chinese medicine, is caused by the stirring of Liver wind in combination with other factors. The stiff tongue can also appear before an attack of wind-stroke, in which case it is a useful prodromal sign together with numbness of the first three fingers of one hand.[2] Extreme internal heat can stir the Liver and give rise to internal wind.

The significance of a stiff tongue was recognized in *Simple Questions:* "When wind enters the body. . .the tongue is stiff."[3] Similarly, the *Classic of Central Treasure* observes, "When Heart and Spleen are attacked by wind, the tongue is stiff and the patient cannot speak."[4] As these passages show, a stiff tongue is never merely a sign of a channel problem, but always reflects disharmony of the internal Organs. It arises either from heat (indicated by a red or dark red tongue) or internal wind (indicated by a tongue of pale or normal color). Thus, as noted by Sun Si-Miao in the *Thousand Ducat Prescriptions*, "If the tongue is stiff and the patient cannot speak, the disease is in the Organs."[5]

Other clinical manifestations will depend on the specific pathology involved. Signs of heat invading the Pericardium include delirium, slurred speech, aphasia, high fever, convulsions and a rapid, overflowing pulse. This is a state of acute disease.

Signs of heat injuring the body fluids vary greatly depending on which Organ is primarily involved. There will, however, be signs and symptoms of malnourished sinews, muscles and channels such as muscle stiffness, cramps, impairment of movement and difficulty in walking.

Signs of blazing Heart fire include insomnia, thirst, a bitter taste in the mouth, irritability, palpitations, mouth ulcers, redness of the face and a rapid, flooding pulse.

Signs of the sequelae of wind-stroke include hemiplegia, asymmetry of the face, slurred speech, muscle stiffness and deviation of the tongue.

FLACCID

A flaccid tongue is flabby and cannot move easily (PLATE 7). In severe cases it has a crumpled look, with many lines on its surface. The flaccid tongue should not be confused with the normal tongue, which is also soft but not as flabby. The normal tongue is also more flexible and mobile than the flaccid tongue.

All types of flaccid tongues are due to a lack of tongue nourishment from deficiency of body fluids. The *Differentiation of Syndromes by Examination of the Tongue* observes, "When the muscles are soft, the tongue is flaccid."[6]

If the tongue is pale and flaccid, it indicates that the Heart and Spleen qi are deficient, and also that the blood is deficient. Not enough fluids and blood reach the tongue, which then becomes flaccid. This condition is primarily caused by an insufficiency of Spleen qi, which fails to produce blood and move fluids. The resulting deficiency of blood affects the Heart (which is always weakened by a deficiency of blood) and therefore the tongue. Deficiency of the Spleen and Heart qi and blood may also lead to malnourishment of the flesh and channels, with resulting weakness of limbs and, in severe cases, atrophy of muscles. Other clinical manifestations include palpitations, insomnia, weak limbs, lassitude, loss of appetite, loose stool, hypersomnia, and a weak pulse.

If the tongue is red and flaccid, it indicates that heat has injured the body fluids. This could involve heat from either excess or deficiency, depending on whether or not there is a tongue coating (PLATE 7). In either case, a flaccid tongue which is also red indicates that the heat is quite intense. The injury to body fluids from heat leads to malnourishment of the sinews and channels, which are deprived of the yin fluids and blood. This may also lead to weakness of the limbs or, in severe cases, atrophy of muscles and impairment of the ability to walk.

If the tongue is red with a coating, this indicates the presence of heat from excess which could be in the Lungs, Heart, Liver or Stomach. (The clinical manifestations of heat in these Organs was previously described.) The most common condition which gives rise to a red and flaccid tongue with coating is heat invading the Lungs. When external heat invades the Lungs and is not properly treated, the heat penetrates into the interior. The heat burns the body fluids and impairs the Lungs' function of dispersing the body fluids and causing them to descend. The clinical manifestations of this condition include a dry cough, or cough with scanty, purulent yellow sputum, nosebleeds, sore throat, dryness of the mouth, fever, restlessness, flaring of the nostrils and a rapid, full and over-flowing pulse.

If the tongue is deep red, flaccid and very dry, it indicates extreme deficiency of Kidney yin leading to severe depletion of body fluids by heat. The deep red color derives from deficiency fire, and the dryness and flaccid quality from an insufficiency of fluids. This condition is very serious. Other clinical signs of Kidney yin deficiency were previously described.

Whatever its type, a flaccid tongue is always due to a deficiency of fluids and malnourishment of the channels. From the perspective of the eight principles iden-tification of patterns, a flaccid tongue always indicates a deficiency condition which, however, can also occur in conjunction with an aspect of excess, such as heat.

LONG

A long tongue is rather thin in its width, although not in its thickness. When extended, a long tongue protrudes from the mouth further than normal so that the root is very clearly visible.

A long tongue generally indicates the presence of heat and will therefore also be red. It is usually associated with heat in the Heart and, from the perspective of Chinese medicine (but not modern biomedicine), indicates a constitutional ten-dency to Heart problems.

If the tongue is long and red and the tip is swollen and redder than the tongue body, the presence of phlegm and fire in the Heart is indicated. A person with this condition will tend to frequently extend and withdraw the tip of their tongue, somewhat in the manner of a snake. Other clinical manifestations include insom-nia, mental restlessness, incoherent speech, uncontrolled laughter, redness of the face, dryness of the mouth, thirst, mouth ulcers, dark yellow urine and a rapid, full and overflowing pulse.

SHORT

A short tongue cannot be fully extended from the mouth and appears to be contracted. There are two basic causes of a short tongue, one from deficiency and the other from excess. A tongue can be short either because internal cold stiffens the sinews and muscles so that the muscles controlling tongue movement cannot extend it, or because excess heat exhausts the body fluids so that the tongue lacks the suppleness to be extended from the mouth.

There are four types of short tongues: pale and short, red and short, deep red, dry and short, and swollen and short.

Pale and Short

A pale, short tongue indicates a deficiency of qi and yang, leading to the for-mation of internal cold, which stiffens and contracts the muscles and sinews.

The tongue is pale from yang deficiency and short from cold that stiffens the tongue muscle. This condition is usually related to deficiency of Spleen or Kidney yang, the signs and symptoms of which were previously described.

Red and Short

A red, short tongue is the result of extreme internal heat which stirs the Liver and gives rise to internal wind. Wind causes contraction and paralysis, thus the short and contracted tongue. This type of tongue is common after an attack of wind-stroke, as well as before, which makes it an important prodromal sign. Besides being short, the tongue will also typically be deviated to one side, which is a further indication of internal wind. (For more information about wind-stroke, refer to the discussion of the deviated tongue below.)

Deep Red, Dry and Short

A deep red, dry and short tongue indicates that extreme heat has injured the body fluids, which then fail to nourish the tongue. The tongue thus cannot be extended. This could be due to Liver heat, the clinical manifestations of which were previously described. If the tongue has no coating and is deep red, dry and short, it indicates that the extreme deficiency of yin fluids prevents the tongue from being extended (PLATE 3).

Swollen and Short

A swollen, short tongue indicates the retention of damp-phlegm in the sinews and muscles, which prevents the tongue from being extended. This is usually due to deficiency of Spleen and/or Lung yang, which fails to transform the fluids. The fluids then accumulate and form damp-phlegm.

CRACKED

A cracked tongue is frequently seen in clinical practice. The cracks on the tongue's surface resemble those that develop in soil after a prolonged period of drought. These cracks can vary greatly in number and depth. They can be barely visible lines or extremely deep fissures. However, sometimes a flaccid tongue can be so soft that it develops a crumpled appearance with lines on its surface; it is important that these lines not be mistaken for cracks.

The clinical significance of cracks depends on the tongue body color, the location of the cracks and their shape and depth. By far the most common cause of cracks is dryness from exhaustion of the body fluids or yin. This condition was described in *A Collection of Tongues and Coatings:* "When the Heart is full . . . the heat cracks the tongue."[7] A common type of cracked tongue has a deep crack in the center reaching to the tip, reflecting hyperactivity of Heart fire.

Most of the cracked tongue types are described in the following passage from the *Guide to Tongue Differentiation:*

A cracked tongue indicates exhaustion of blood. The fewer and more superficial the cracks, the milder the disease. The deeper and more numerous the cracks, the more serious the disease. Horizontal cracks indicate yin deficiency; if there are cracks like ice floes, it indicates yin deficiency from old age. If the tongue is pale and has cracks, it indicates Spleen deficiency with retention of dampness... If the whole tongue is deep red without coating and there are short horizontal cracks, it indicates yin deficiency with depletion of body fluids... Short, irregular cracks indicate Stomach dryness with depletion of fluids and heat from excess inside.[8]

Long Horizontal Cracks

Long horizontal cracks generally indicate deficiency of yin and are commonly (but not exclusively) found in red tongues without coating (ILLUSTRATION 6-9). They may also be observed in tongues of normal color, in which case the condition is less serious than it would be if the tongue were red and without coating. If the tongue is red, the yin deficiency stems from the Kidneys. If the tongue color is normal, the deficiency stems from the Stomach and/or Lungs.

Short Horizontal Cracks

The clinical significance of short horizontal cracks is similar to that of long horizontal ones (ILLUSTRATION 6-10).

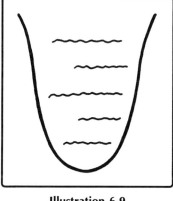

Illustration 6-9

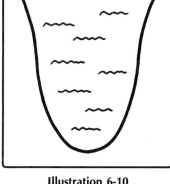

Illustration 6-10

They also indicate yin deficiency, but are more commonly found on a red tongue without coating. Short horizontal cracks also indicate heat stemming from yin deficiency.

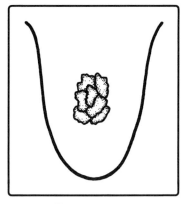

Illustration 6-11

Cracks Resembling Ice Floes

Cracks that resemble ice floes (PLATE 13 & ILLUSTRATION 6-11) are frequently seen among the elderly. They simply indicate a condition of yin deficiency from old age. It is very common for the elderly to develop yin deficiency because the energy of the Kidneys becomes depleted as we grow older. In this case the tongue may or may not be red. If the tongue has a normal color, the cracks do not have much clinical significance. If, however, the tongue is red and without coating, the cracks indicate an advanced stage of yin deficiency from heat. Persons so afflicted will probably suffer from night sweats and pain in the joints stemming from the exhaustion of the yin fluids, which fail to nourish the sinews and channels. This type of tongue is common in women experiencing menopausal problems.

Irregular Cracks

Short, irregular cracks (PLATE 25 & ILLUSTRATION 6-12) indicate deficiency of Stomach yin. The Stomach is the origin of fluids in the body and a malfunction of the

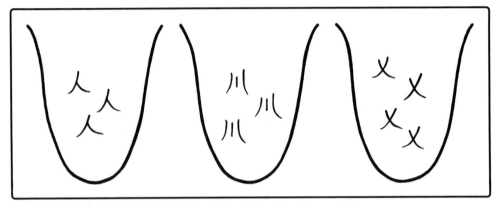

Illustration 6-12

Stomach often leads to a deficiency of body fluids. This may be the very first stage of yin deficiency. In this case the tongue will be of normal color.

Transverse Cracks on the Sides

Transverse cracks (PLATES 34, 57 & ILLUSTRATION 6-13) can occur on a tongue of normal color. They always indicate a long-standing condition of Spleen qi or Spleen yin deficiency. The cracks are on the sides and usually only within the central third of the tongue. If the sides are cracked and also wet and slightly foamy, this reflects a long-standing condition of Spleen qi deficiency. Spleen qi, in this case, is unable to transform and transport the fluids, which then accumulate on the tongue.

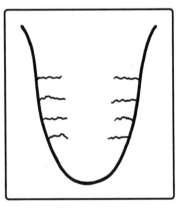

Illustration 6-13

If the tongue is dry, or if only the edges are dry, transverse cracks indicate Spleen yin deficiency. The manifestations of Spleen yin deficiency are dry mouth with no desire to drink, a feeling of heat in the face, dry lips, dry stools, poor appetite, abdominal discomfort and tiredness. Dry lips, in particular, are a key symptom in this pattern.

Vertical Crack in the Center

A broad, shallow crack in the midline and within the central third of the tongue (PLATE 25 & ILLUSTRATION 6-14) indicates deficiency of Stomach qi in a tongue of normal color with a coating. In a tongue of normal color without a coating, it indicates deficiency of Stomach yin. In the latter case it signifies that the yin deficiency affects only the Stomach and has not yet reached the Kidneys.

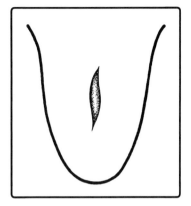

Illustration 6-14

If a crack such as this appears with a sticky, yellow, dry and rough-looking coating inside, it indicates the presence of phlegm-fire in the Stomach. A patient so afflicted may also complain of excessive appetite with a feeling of fullness after eating, dryness of the mouth, thirst with a preference for drinking in small sips, bleeding gums, vomiting, and, in severe cases, vomiting blood. It also often denotes the possibility of mental illness, such as manic-depression.

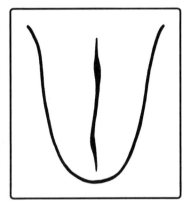

Illustration 6-15

Long Vertical Crack in the Center

A long, deep vertical crack in the midline of the tongue reaching to the tip or just short of the tip (PLATES 7, 11, 17, 26 & ILLUSTRATION 6-15) is always related to the Heart. Its significance depends on the tongue body color and the depth of the crack. Generally, the deeper the crack, the more serious the condition. There are three possibilities: normal color, red with redder tip, and red with no coating.

NORMAL COLOR

In a tongue of normal color, the long crack in the midline simply indicates a slight constitutional weakness of the Heart and is not necessarily a sign of disease (PLATE 17). Of course, indications on the tongue should be correlated with other signs. This slight weakness is indicated if the tongue body color is normal, the Heart pulse only slightly weak, but the other pulses generally good, and there are no Heart symptoms.

RED WITH REDDER TIP

If the tongue body color is red and the tip is redder still, the midline crack indicates the presence of Heart fire (PLATE 7). In this case, there is a constitutional weakness of the Heart and also Heart fire. The Heart fire is usually caused by deep emotional problems. The tip may also be swollen and have red points.

RED WITH NO COATING

If the tongue body color is red and the tongue has no coating, the midline crack indicates the presence of deficiency heat affecting the Heart (PLATES 11 & 26). There is a general condition of yin deficiency of the Kidneys leading to the for-

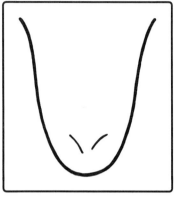

Illustration 6-16

mation of deficiency heat in the Heart (water failing to control fire). This condition can also arise from long-standing emotional problems and extended periods of overwork.

Transverse Cracks Behind the Tip

One or two small transverse cracks at a 45 degree angle slanting toward the midline, located just behind the tongue tip in the area corresponding to the Lungs (PLATE 59 & ILLUSTRATION 6-16), usually indicates such prior Lung diseases as childhood pneumonia, whooping cough or pulmonary tuberculosis. A present tendency to Lung yin deficiency is also indicated.

Deep Central Crack with Other Small Cracks

When there is an extremely deep midline crack with other small cracks branching out from or scattered on the tongue, and the body color is deep red with no coating (PLATE 24 & ILLUSTRATION 6-17), this always indicates heat from extreme deficiency of Kidney yin and great dryness of the body. It is often seen in cases of kidney stones, although not all kidney stone cases will present with this type of tongue. This configuration may reflect deep and long-standing emotional problems as well as over-work, stress and/or poor eating habits.

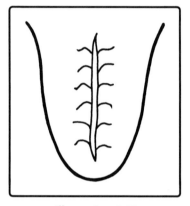

Illustration 6-17

LOOSE

A loose tongue hangs outside the mouth when it is extended, and is difficult to retract. It may drip with saliva. The clinical significance of this tongue type depends on other aspects of its consistency and on the color of the tongue body.

If the tongue is loose, stiff and dry, it indicates the retention of interior heat from excess, normally of the Liver and Heart. This tongue may be found in cases of wind-stroke from Liver wind, and fire affecting the Heart and giving rise to Heart fire. The tongue is stiff because of the wind, and dry because of the heat.

If the tongue is loose, deep red and long, and the patient is unconscious, delirious or laughing uncontrollably, it indicates the retention of phlegm-fire in the Heart. This is a case of phlegm-fire clouding the Heart, which is also called "misting over the consciousness."

If the tongue is loose and numb, it indicates qi deficiency, usually of the Heart. If a child's tongue is totally loose so that it cannot be withdrawn at all, it indicates a serious collapse of Heart qi.

DEVIATED

A tongue that deviates to one side when extended is usually (but not always) found in conjunction with asymmetry of the face (PLATE 51). A deviated tongue generally indicates the presence of wind, which can be external or internal.

External wind can invade the channels of the face and cause facial paralysis, with deviation of the mouth, inability to raise the eyebrows and sometimes deviation of the tongue when it is extended.

Internal wind has an entirely different origin and nature. It usually derives from deficiency of Kidney yin and hyperactivity of Liver yang, but it may also result from deficiency of Liver blood. The clinical signs of internal wind are tremor, tics and spasms, dizziness, numbness and deviation of the tongue. Wind-stroke is always associated with internal wind, although there are other pathological factors involved. Internal wind may affect only the channels, in which case there is no loss of consciousness, but merely an often-passing impairment of movement in a limb and numbness. When internal wind affects the Organs there will be sudden loss of consciousness and other disturbances, followed by hemiplegia and asymmetry of the face. In either case, the tongue can be deviated.

The *Guide to Tongue Differentiation* summarizes the wind patterns associated with a deviated tongue:

> If the tongue is purplish-red and deviated, it signifies Liver wind. If it is pale and deviated, it signifies wind-stroke. If it is deviated and there is facial paralysis, it signifies [external] wind invading the channels.[9]

Deviation of the tongue may also be caused by deficiency, in contrast to the excessive conditions (or deficiency complicated by excess) previously described. For example, when there is severe Heart qi or Heart blood deficiency, there is not enough blood and qi reaching the tongue. The tongue muscles become slack and the tongue deviates when extended.

Rong Chun-Nian (1800–1881) described the tongue as the "tendon of the brain" and correlated certain pathological colors of the tongue with brain conditions such as "brain heat."[10] Rong's description of the tongue as the "tendon of the brain" is corroborated by Western anatomy, as the motor nerve to the tongue is the 12th cranial nerve. This nerve can be affected by lesions in its connections between the motor cortex and the brain stem, leading to a deviated tongue.

NUMB

A numb tongue is always directly attributable to a failure of the nutritive qi and blood in reaching and nourishing the tongue. If the tongue is periodically loose and numb, it indicates Heart blood deficiency in which the blood of the Heart does not reach and nourish the tongue. If the tongue is numb and there is dizziness and blurred vision, it indicates internal movement of Liver wind.

A special case is presented when the tongue has a slippery coating, the corners of the mouth are numb and there is copious production of sputum. This indicates the presence of wind-phlegm.

MOVING

A moving tongue is one which moves slowly from one side to the other when extended, or moves without stopping and can only be extended to show a small part of the tongue body. This tongue indicates the presence of internal wind generated by the Liver, which may be due to various etiologies. It is often seen in patients after cerebral vascular accidents. When Liver wind is accompanied by Heart fire the moving tongue will also be deep red and dry. The addition of Spleen heat is indicated by a moving tongue that is red, swollen and dry on its sides. Although uncommon, both Heart fire and Spleen heat may occur together.

QUIVERING

It is important to distinguish a moving from a quivering tongue. The movements of a moving tongue are slow but with large amplitude. A quivering tongue, on the other hand, is characterized by rapid movements of small amplitude when extended.

The clinical significance of a quivering tongue depends on the color of the tongue body. A quivering tongue is most often pale or pale red. This indicates qi and blood deficiency, usually accompanied by Spleen yang deficiency. If the quivering tongue is red and dry, it indicates extreme heat inside, which gives rise to internal wind. A quivering, deep red and flapping tongue signifies Liver heat toxin generating internal wind. A quivering tongue accompanied by aphasia or dysphasia indicates the collapse of Heart and Spleen qi.

A quivering, pale and flaccid tongue indicates the collapse of the yang from profuse and protracted sweating. In this situation the sinews and channels lose the nourishment of the yang qi and the moistening of the body fluids.

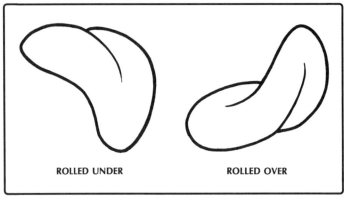

ROLLED UNDER   ROLLED OVER

Illustration 6-18

ROLLED

The rolled tongue has a tip which either rolls over or under (ILLUSTRATION 6-18). It always indicates heat in the Heart. When the tongue is rolled under, there is deficiency heat. When the tip is rolled over, there is heat from excess.

TOOTH-MARKED

A tooth-marked tongue (also referred to as a "scalloped tongue") has clear indentations on its sides (ILLUSTRATION 6-19). This is usually caused by Spleen qi deficiency. The tongue body color is commonly pale or normal.

A survey in China of 425 patients with tooth-marked tongues found that 345 suffered from qi or yang deficiency.[11]

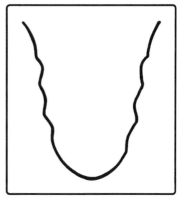

Illustration 6-19

ULCERATED

Swollen, painful red ulcers with red rims on the surface of the tongue usually signify Heart fire blazing upward. If the ulcers have a white edge, Heart heat from Kidney yin deficiency may be indicated. If the ulcers are underneath the tongue body, they are caused by extreme heat in the Spleen and Kidneys that is exhausting the body fluids.

SORE-COVERED

A sore-covered tongue will have sores like rice grains scattered on the four corners of both its upper and lower surfaces. The sores may or may not be painful. They usually indicate heat in the upper burner and are most frequently attributed to heat toxin in the Heart channel. If the sores are convex and painful, they are caused by heat toxin in the Heart blazing upward. If the sores are concave and painless, they are due to yin deficiency of the lower burner, with heat from the deficiency floating upward.

SUMMARY

Examination of the shape of the tongue body follows examination of the body color. The importance of the body shape is two-fold:

- It provides an indication of the severity of the condition. For example, a pale tongue may indicate blood deficiency, but if it is pale and thin it signifies that the blood deficiency is severe.

- It provides an indication of the duration of the condition. For example, a red tongue without coating indicates yin deficiency, but if it is also thin it signifies that the yin deficiency is of long duration. Both of these characteristics are important in determining the prognosis and estimating the duration of treatment.

Except in rare cases, the clinical significance of the body shape is always subordinate to that of the body color. By this is meant that one cannot talk about the significance of a thin body without relating it to the body color.

From the perspective of the eight principles identification of patterns, the tongue body shape provides a clear expression of deficiency or excess. Examples of deficient body shapes include thin, flaccid, cracked and tooth-marked. Examples of excess body shapes include swollen, stiff, long and moving. Other types of body shapes (such as short, loose, deviated, numb, quivering, rolled, ulcerated and with sores) may indicate either deficiency or excess depending on the color of the tongue body.

NOTES

1. Cao Bing-Zhang, *A Guide to Tongue Differentiation.* Cited in Beijing College of Traditional Chinese Medicine, *Tongue Diagnosis in Chinese Medicine (Zhong yi she zhen)* (Beijing: People's Medical Publishing House, 1976), p. 32.

2. Su Xin-Ming, personal communication.

3. *Yellow Emperor's Inner Classic: Simple Questions (Huang di nei jing su wen)* (Beijing: People's Medical Publishing House, 1963), chap. 74, p. 512.

4. Attributed to Hua *Tuo, Classic of the Central Treasure (Zhong cang jing)* (Han dynasty). Cited in *Tongue Diagnosis in Chinese Medicine,* p. 33.

5. Sun Si-Miao, *Thousand Ducat Prescriptions,* chap. 22. Cited in *Tongue Diagnosis in Chinese Medicine,* p. 33.

6. Liang Te-Yan, *Differentiation of Syndromes by Examination of the Tongue.* Cited in *Tongue Diagnosis in Chinese Medicine,* p. 26.

7. Fu Song-Yuan, *A Collection of Tongues and Coatings.* Cited in *Tongue Diagnosis in Chinese Medicine,* p. 26.

8. Cao Bing-Zhang, *A Guide to Tongue Differentiation.* Cited in *Tongue Diagnosis in Chinese Medicine,* pp. 33-34.

9. *A Guide to Tongue Differentiation.* Cited in *Tongue Diagnosis in Chinese Medicine,* pp. 34-35.

10. Hu Ming-Can, "Rong Chun-Nian's Tongue Diagnosis." *Journal of Traditional Chinese Medicine (Zhong yi za zhi)* 30, no.12 (1989): 13.

11. Qian Xin-Ru, "Analysis of Clinical Observation of Patients with Tooth-marked Tongue." *Journal of Traditional Chinese Medicine* 32, no. 1 (1991): 33.

TABLE OF TONGUE BODY SHAPE

BODY SHAPE	CLINICAL SIGNIFICANCE
Thin	Deficient blood (pale body) Deficient yin (red body)
Swollen	Spleen and/or Kidney yang deficiency with dampness Damp-heat in Stomach and Spleen Heart and Stomach heat (red body) Alcoholic toxin (red body) Toxin
Swollen edges	Spleen qi deficiency
Swollen sides	Ascendant Liver yang or Liver fire
Swollen tip	Heart fire blazing (red body) Heart qi deficiency (normal color)
Swollen between tip and center	Lung qi deficiency with retention of phlegm
Swollen along central crack	Heart fire blazing (red body) Heart qi deficiency (normal color)
Half swollen	Weakness of the channels
Partly swollen on side	Deficiency or stagnation of qi in chest
Half surface swollen	Lung qi deficiency
Hammer-shaped	Stomach, Spleen and Kidney deficiency
Stiff	Exterior heat invading Pericardium (red or dark red body) Heat injuring body fluids (red body) Blazing Heart fire Internal wind (normal color)
Flaccid	Exhausted qi and blood (pale body) Extreme heat injuring fluids (red body) Kidney yin deficiency with heat (deep red body)
Long	Blazing Heart fire Phlegm-fire in Heart
Short	Spleen yang deficiency, internal cold (pale body) Heat stirring Liver wind (red body) Insufficiency of body fluids due to heat from excess (red body with coating)

BODY SHAPE	CLINICAL SIGNIFICANCE
Short, cont.	Deficiency heat (red body without coating) Spleen yang deficiency with dampness and phlegm (pale body with slippery coating)
Cracked	Horizontal cracks: yin deficiency Cracks like ice floes: yin deficiency from old age Irregular cracks: stomach yin deficiency Transverse cracks on sides: Spleen qi deficiency Vertical cracks in center: Heart yin deficiency or blazing Heart fire Transverse cracks behind tip: Lung yin deficiency Very deep central crack with other small cracks: Kidney yin deficiency with heat
Loose	Interior excess heat (red body) Phlegm-fire clouding Heart (red body with slippery coating) Heart qi deficiency (pale body)
Deviated	Exterior wind invading channels (normal color) Interior Liver wind (red or normal color) Heart qi deficiency (pale body)
Numb	Heart blood deficiency (pale body) Liver wind (red or normal color) Wind-phlegm (slippery coating)
Moving	Heart fire and internal wind (red body) Spleen heat with exhaustion of body fluids (red and dry body)
Quivering	Spleen qi deficiency (pale body) Extreme heat generating internal wind (red body) Collapse of Heart and Spleen qi (pale body) Collapse of yang (pale and thin body)
Rolled	Heat from excess (tip rolled over) Deficiency heat (tip rolled under)
Tooth-marked	Spleen qi deficiency
Ulcerated	Blazing Heart fire (red body) Heart heat from Kidney yin deficiency (red and peeled body) Spleen and Kidney heat (red body)
Sore-covered	Heat toxin in Heart channel (red body) Deficiency heat (red and peeled body)

7
Tongue Coating

The tongue coating (also called fur or moss) consists of the tips of the papillae, which are epithelial projections on the dorsum of the tongue. There are five types of papillae, but those which constitute the coating are mostly the filiform ones.

From the perspective of Chinese medicine, the tongue coating is a physiological by-product of the Stomach's digestion of food and fluids.

Examination of the tongue coating is a very important aspect of tongue diagnosis in Chinese medicine. It is so much a part of the routine examination in China that the practitioner, when asking the patient to show his or her tongue, will often say, "Let's look at your tongue coating" (kàn kàn shé tāi).

PHYSIOLOGY OF TONGUE COATING

The digestive function depends on the Spleen's transformation and transportation of food, and on the Stomach's fermenting and ripening of food. The digestive process is seen in Chinese medicine as one of bubbling, fermenting ("rotting and ripening") and boiling, as in a cauldron. This process is associated with dampness and what the ancient Chinese called "turbidity." In the process of digestion, a small amount comes up to the tongue and forms the coating.

The tongue coating is thus the result of a physiological process and its presence on the tongue indicates the proper functioning of the Spleen and, primarily, the Stomach. A normal tongue *should* have a coating. Chinese texts say that the tongue coating is a manifestation of Stomach qi and that a healthy person should have a thin coating like grass growing from the soil.

The normal tongue coating is thin, white and slightly moist. It is thin because only a small amount of turbidity flows up from the Stomach as a by-product of digestion. If the coating is unduly thick, it indicates excessive turbidity in the

Stomach or improper functioning of the digestive process. If the coating is too thin or altogether absent, it indicates that the Stomach's digestive function is severely impaired.

A tongue coating is too thick when it covers the tongue surface entirely so that the tongue body cannot be seen beneath it. As described in the *Interpretation of the Discussion of Cold-induced Disorders*,[1] a tongue coating of normal thickness will be sparse enough for the tongue body to be seen, in the way that the earth can be seen between the blades of newly-sprouted grass. To extend this analogy, a coating that is too thin is like a bare patch of lawn.

The Stomach is the origin of fluids. A slightly moist coating indicates a basically healthy state of the Stomach fluids. The Stomach "fears" dryness and when it becomes dry the supply of fluids to the entire body is affected. At the other extreme, if the Stomach does not digest food properly and food and fluids accumulate, the tongue coating may become too wet or even slippery.

The practitioner needs to observe the *distribution* of the coating. Normally, there is a subtle progression of coating thickness in different areas of the tongue surface. The coating should be thinnest on the tip and edges of the tongue, slightly thicker in the center, and even thicker on the root. Since the coating reflects the condition of the Stomach, it is only natural that a slightly thicker coating should be found on the central surface of the tongue in the area corresponding to the Stomach itself. The root of the tongue corresponds to the Intestines, which are involved in the Stomach's digestive processes. Because the Intestines process impure substances, this natural turbidity will be reflected as a thicker coating on the root.

CLINICAL SIGNIFICANCE OF TONGUE COATING

From very early times, and particularly since the Han dynasty's *Discussion of Cold-induced Disorders*, Chinese medical literature has noted the relationship between changes in tongue coating and pathological changes in the human body. As one medical text observed, "The tongue coating originates from the evaporation of Stomach qi. Because the five yin Organs receive qi from the Stomach, one can know from the coating the conditions of deficiency or excess and heat or cold [of all the Organs]."[2]

Since the tongue coating is formed as a by-product of the digestive process, its thickness, consistency and color all provide an immediate and accurate indication of the functional state of the Stomach and Spleen. However, the coating also reflects the condition of other Organs such as the Kidneys, Intestines, Liver, Gallbladder, Bladder and Lungs. The particular relationships between certain tongue coatings and pathological conditions of these Organs will be discussed later in this chapter.

Although secondary to the Stomach and Spleen, the Kidneys also play an important role in the formation of the coating. One of the Kidneys' functions is to "evaporate" the body's fluids, sending them upward. Part of the product of this evaporation process flows up to the tongue where it contributes, together with the products of the Stomach and Spleen, to the formation of the tongue coating. A total lack of coating therefore indicates not only a Stomach, but also a Kidney deficiency.

Apart from reflecting the condition of various Organs, the tongue coating is extremely important because it shows the strength and depth of various pathogenic factors (wind-cold, wind-heat, dampness, etc.). This is probably the primary clinical significance of the coating, the observation of which is vital in acute, externally-contracted diseases.

The tongue coating can also provide information about a variety of internal conditions such as retention of food, dampness, phlegm, heat and cold. Finally, the tongue coating can give an immediate indication of the state of the body fluids.

From the perspective of the eight principles identification of patterns, examination of the tongue coating allows the practitioner to differentiate between deficiency and excess, hot and cold, interior and exterior, and yin and yang conditions.

TONGUE COATING IN ACUTE, EXTERNALLY-CONTRACTED DISEASES

Examination of tongue coating is particularly important in acute, externally-contracted diseases because the thickness and distribution of the coating can provide an immediate and accurate indication of the strength and depth of the pathogenic factor. This is very useful in prognosis.

The thicker the tongue coating, the greater the intensity of the pathogenic factor. This rule, however, only applies in the context of externally-contracted diseases; not every thick coating indicates the presence of an external pathogenic factor. The rule simply means that, if there really is such a factor present, the thickness of the coating is proportionate to its intensity.

A clinical example will illustrate this rule. In an external attack of wind-cold invading the exterior portion of the body the tongue coating will be thin, white and probably slightly wet. Its thinness reflects the onset of the disease when the pathogenic factor (wind-cold) has only just penetrated the body. It will be white because it is caused by wind-cold (as opposed to wind-heat) and slightly wet because of the impairment of the Lungs' ability to disperse fluids, which then accumulate on the tongue. If this condition is not treated properly and the wind-cold is not expelled, it may penetrate deeper and become stronger. This will be reflected as a thicker tongue coating. If the wind-cold changes into heat (a common occurrence), the coating will change from white to yellow.

The distribution of the coating as well as its thickness is closely related to changes in the pathological condition and depth of the pathogenic factor's penetration in externally-contracted diseases. To illustrate this, we may expand upon the clinical situation described above. At the onset of an attack of wind-cold upon the exterior portion of the body the coating may be more concentrated in the front third of the tongue, or possibly on its edges. Both of these areas correspond to the exterior. If the pathogenic factor penetrates deeper, the coating may move from the front third or the edges of the tongue to its central surface. It will, at this point, become thicker. The movement and thickening of the coating indicate both that the pathogenic factor has moved to the interior and that it has become stronger. The coating may also change from white to yellow, indicating that wind-cold on the exterior has transformed into heat in the interior.

The relationship between the tongue coating and external pathogenic factors will be discussed in further detail in this chapter. We will begin with a brief description of the tongue coatings which may be expected to occur in attacks of the most common external pathogenic factors.

Wind-Cold

The tongue coating will be thin in the initial stages and white, reflecting the presence of cold. It may also be slightly wet or slightly slippery, reflecting the impairment of the Lungs' fluid-dispersing function by the obstruction of wind-cold in the exterior (skin and muscles). The coating may be more concentrated in the front third or on the edges of the tongue because the wind-cold is located in the exterior of the body. Other clinical manifestations include headache, a stiff neck, pains in the body, the presence or absence of sweat and absence of thirst, pronounced chills and slight fever, aversion to cold and a tight, floating pulse.

Wind-Heat

The tongue coating will be thin in the initial stages and yellow, reflecting the presence of heat. It may also be slightly dry because heat dries up the body fluids. As in the case of wind-cold, the coating may be more concentrated in the front third or on the edges of the tongue. In some cases, especially in children, there may also be red points in those same areas, reflecting the special virulence of the pathogenic factor. (The presence of red points in the context of externally-contracted diseases is discussed in chapter 6.) Other clinical manifestations include headache, sore throat, swollen tonsils, pains in the body, thirst, slight sweating, slight chills and pronounced fever and a floating, rapid pulse.

Heat

This is also called "summer heat" in Chinese medicine, which, contrary to other pathogenic factors which can occur in any season, only occurs in summertime. In the initial stages, the tongue coating will be thin and yellow, reflecting the presence of heat. It will also be dry because heat injures the body fluids. Other clinical manifestations include aversion to heat, profuse sweating, headache, dry lips, thirst and an overflowing, rapid pulse.

Cold

External cold can attack the Stomach, Womb, and Intestines directly without first manifesting changes in the exterior portions of the body. The tongue coating in each of these cases will be thick, reflecting the intensity of the pathogenic factor that is already in the interior. The coating will also be white because of the cold, and possibly wet, indicating the obstruction of normal fluid movement by cold. It is important to stress that although the cold is of external origin it penetrates the interior of the body directly. It is thereafter manifested as internal cold. This disorder may be contrasted with an invasion by wind-cold which goes through the exterior of the body before penetrating to the interior.

Clinical manifestations will vary according to the location of the cold. The primary sign will be pain, either epigastric (with nausea and vomiting) or abdominal (with diarrhea), depending upon the location of the cold in the Stomach, Intestines or Womb. The pulse will be slow and tight in all three cases. In women, abdominal pain and diarrhea may occur during menstruation, accompanied by intense dysmenorrhea and clots in the menstrual blood.

Dampness

External dampness can attack the Stomach, Intestines or muscles and channels. The tongue coating will be thick because of the dampness, and both greasy and slippery, reflecting the obstruction by dampness of the transformation and transportation of fluids.

Other clinical manifestations will vary according to the location of the dampness but usually include a feeling of heaviness, abdominal distension, stuffiness of the chest, loose stools, and a slippery, full pulse.

TONGUE COATING AND THE EIGHT PRINCIPLES

The tongue coating can provide an accurate indication of the nature of the disease from the perspective of the eight principles identification of patterns. This is particularly true in cases of acute, externally-contracted diseases.

Exterior

The exterior portion of the body (skin, muscles and channels) is reflected either in the front third or on the edges of the tongue. In exterior conditions the tongue coating may be more concentrated in these areas.

Interior

The interior condition of the body is reflected on the central surface of the tongue. The tongue coating may be concentrated on the edges of the tongue in the initial stage of invasion by an external pathogenic factor (ILLUSTRATION 7-1).

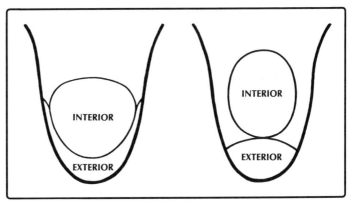

Illustration 7-1

If it is not expelled, the pathogenic factor may penetrate deeper to the Organs, in which case the coating on the central surface will become thicker. (It will also probably — though not necessarily — become yellow.) This progression occurs only in the context of the penetration of external factors to the interior. The tongue coating, of course, also reflects chronic internal conditions, in which case a thick coating in the center might indicate retention of food or dampness in the Stomach.

Deficiency

Deficiency conditions are reflected on the tongue by an absence or insufficiency of coating. Insufficient coating, or a coating without root, indicates deficient Stomach qi. The complete absence of coating when the tongue body color is red indicates deficiency of both Stomach and Kidney yin. If there is no coating and the tongue body is pale, deficient blood is indicated. If there is no coating and the tongue body color is normal, deficient Stomach yin is the diagnosis.

Excess

Excess conditions are always indicated by a thick tongue coating. (A condition of excess may, however, be associated with one of deficiency.) A thick coating indicates the presence of a pathogenic factor battling with the body's energies, which are still sufficiently strong to resist the attack. Whether or not there is a coating is often crucial in differentiating between conditions of deficiency and excess. For example, if the tongue body color is red or deep red the presence of a coating (whether it is thick or thin) indicates excess heat, while the absence of a coating indicates deficiency heat.

Heat

The color of the tongue coating in heat patterns will be yellow.

Cold

The color of the tongue coating in cold patterns will be white.

Yang

The tongue coating is not an important factor in diagnosing yang deficiency, which is indicated by a pale tongue body color. If deficiency of yang leads to the accumulation of dampness, the tongue coating will be thick, white and slippery.

Yin

Yin deficiency is indicated by an absence of tongue coating. A normal tongue body color in this case means a deficiency of Stomach yin, while a red or deep red body color signifies Kidney yin deficiency.

TONGUE COATING PROPER

With these general principles in mind, we may now consider the various types of tongue coatings in detail, distinguishing first between tongue coating proper and tongue coating color. By tongue coating proper is meant the coating's texture, distribution, thickness, moisture and greasiness. The following aspects of tongue coating proper will be discussed:

- Coating with or without root
- The presence or absence of coating
- Coating thickness
- Coating distribution
- Coating moisture
- Moldy or greasy coatings

Coating With or Without Root

The normal tongue coating has root, i.e., it is closely attached to the tongue surface. It grows out of it much like grass grows from the soil. The coating is hard, firmly adhering to the tongue body. It is also thin, uniformly distributed and cannot be scraped or wiped off. The question of whether or not the tongue coating has root is of extreme importance in clinical practice. It is also important that this not be confused with the question of whether the coating is thin or thick. A coating with root can be thick or thin, and so can a coating without root.

A coating without root looks patchy. It appears to be resting on the surface of the tongue rather than growing out of it. It can easily be wiped or scraped off (PLATES 5, 13, 20, 31, 57 & 59). In severe cases the coating without root may look like powder, snow or salt (PLATES 19 & 23).

A coating loses its root when the Stomach, Spleen and Kidney functions are impaired, i.e., when the Stomach is not transforming and "ripening" the food, the Spleen is not separating the essences of food and the Kidneys are not "evaporating" the fluids upward. When all of these functions are impaired, the proper amount of turbidity does not reach the tongue and does not form a coating. The already-established coating stays on the tongue, but no new coating is formed. The old coating loses its root and floats on the tongue surface. Eventually, it will come off entirely and the tongue surface will be peeled. A coating without root always suggests the possibility that the coating may come off entirely, signifying a worsening of the condition.

The clinical significance of a coating with root depends on its thickness. A thin coating with root indicates a healthy condition of the Stomach and Spleen and is therefore normal. A thick coating with root indicates the presence of a pathogenic factor. The thicker the coating, the stronger the factor. A thick coating with root also means that the body's energies are intact and are fighting the pathogenic factor. This is a pattern of excess.

The clinical significance of a coating without root is independent of its thickness. Whether thin or thick, such a coating always indicates a weakening of the

Stomach, Spleen and Kidneys, and hence a weakening of the body's energies. This is a pattern of deficiency.

One particular kind of coating without root is found on the tongue when one awakens; it disappears after breakfast. This indicates a mild weakness of Stomach qi. A coating without root can also be due to an overdose of herbal medicine used to tonify the Kidney yang or Kidney yin (either an excess of cooling medicines which injure the Kidney yang, or of warming medicines which injure the Kidney yin). Antibiotics can also cause the coating to lose its root.

It is instructive to compare the relative seriousness of a coating with or without root in the pathological development of a disease. In the initial and middle stages of an illness, a thick coating with root is more serious than a coating without root. In these stages the condition is characterized by the presence of a pathogenic factor struggling with the body's energies. A thick coating with root signifies that the pathogenic factors are quite strong. It is important to stress, however, that this concept only applies in the initial and middle stages of an externally-contracted disease when the purpose of treatment is to reduce the pathogenic factors.

In the late stage of a disease, a thick coating without root is more serious than a coating with root. The later stages of disease are characterized by a weakening of the body's energies; the emphasis in treatment is therefore on strengthening the body's energies rather than reducing the pathogenic factors. A coating without root, indicating a serious weakening of the body's energies, is therefore a more serious sign than is a coating with root.

To summarize, a coating without root always indicates a condition of deficiency and a weakening of the body's energies. Specifically, a condition of Stomach qi, Stomach yin or possibly Kidney yin deficiency is indicated.

On the other hand, a thick coating with root always indicates a condition of excess in which there is some pathogenic factor at work, but also in which the body's energies are relatively intact.

A particular type of coating without root is that seen in "geographic" tongues (PLATES 44, 57 & 59). From a Western anatomical perspective, geographic tongues are characterized by a loss of filiform papillae and hyperemia. From a Chinese perspective, these tongues are peeled in patches, which have quite well-defined contours. The coating in the non-peeled areas is without root. Although this tongue can be constitutional and is regarded by some as having no clinical significance, it does, in my opinion, always indicate Stomach yin deficiency, whether constitutional or not. In modern biomedicine, this type of tongue is frequently associated with autoimmune diseases (such as rheumatoid arthritis and systemic lupus erythematosus); there is also an association with a past history or family history of asthma, atopic eczema and allergic rhinitis with raised levels of IgE.[3]

Presence or Absence of Coating

The change in the coating over the course of a disease is an important factor in making a proper diagnosis and prognosis. It is particularly important to recognize those cases in which the coating disappears entirely, and those in which it appears and builds up rather suddenly.

If in the course of a disease the tongue coating suddenly disappears (even if only partially), it indicates that the Stomach yin is becoming exhausted and that the condition is taking a sudden turn for the worse. This is true whether the coating disappears suddenly or slowly, but it is all the more serious if it disappears suddenly. In the latter situation, measures must be taken to treat and tonify the Stomach and Kidney yin quickly and vigorously. For example, the sudden, partial disappearance of coating in a patient with cancer may indicate a metastasis to another organ. This can be correlated to the area of the tongue where the coating has disappeared; e.g., if it is on one side, it might be the liver.

On the other hand, if in the course of a disease there is no tongue coating and one suddenly appears, it indicates that there is turbid dampness in the Stomach, or that pathogenic (interior) heat is increasing. Plates 52 and 53 were taken at a three-day interval and clearly show the sudden appearance of a thick yellow coating in the Lung area on a previously peeled tongue.

It must be emphasized that this rule applies only if the coating appears suddenly, i.e., in the course of a few days. If a tongue at first has lost its coating, but the coating reappears slowly, the restoration and recovery of Stomach qi is indicated. This is a very favorable prognostic sign (PLATES 57 & 58).

In chronic conditions tending to yin deficiency, the coating disappears very gradually: absence of coating is always a certain indication of yin deficiency. Because the coating reflects the state of the Stomach, it follows that yin deficiency always starts with Stomach yin deficiency. Or, to put it differently, in yin deficiency the Stomach is always involved. Illustration 7-2 shows the possible stages from a tongue with a normal rooted coating to one that is totally peeled and red. Of course, such progression only describes the most common stages seen in practice, and many deviations from this progression may occur. The following six basic stages (plus one variation) can be identified:

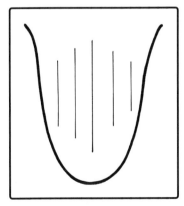

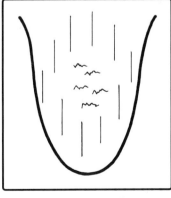

1. The normal tongue has a thin, white coating with root.

2. The coating starts to become rootless in the center, indicating Stomach-qi deficiency.

Illlustration 7-2a   **Illustration 7-2b**

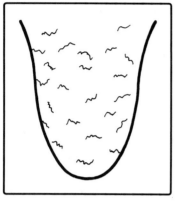

Illustration 7-2c

3. The coating becomes rootless all over, indicating more serious Stomach qi deficiency.

4. The center loses its coating entirely (i.e., becomes peeled), while the remainder of the tongue has a rootless coating, indicating Stomach yin deficiency.

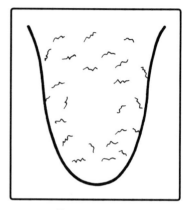

Illustration 7-2d

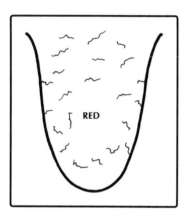

Illustration 7-2e

5. A possible variation of the above tongue is when the center becomes red, indicating Stomach yin deficiency with deficiency heat (PLATES 12 & 20).

6. The tongue becomes peeled all over, losing all its coating (with or without a Stomach crack), indicating more severe Stomach yin deficiency (ILLUSTRATIONS 7-2f & 7-2g and PLATE 25).

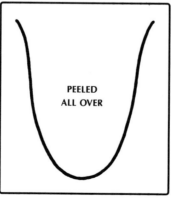

Illustration 7-2f

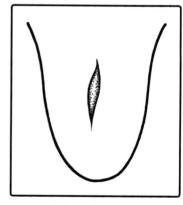

Illustration 7-2g

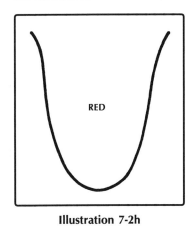

Illustration 7-2h

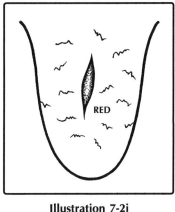

Illustration 7-2i

7. The tongue is peeled all over and red (with or without a Stomach crack), indicating both Stomach- and Kidney-yin deficiency leading to heat (ILLUSTRATIONS 7-2h & 7-2i and PLATES 13, 24 & 59).

Coating Thickness

A thick coating always signifies the presence of a pathogenic factor, and therefore a condition of excess. The relative thickness of the coating gives an immediate and accurate indication of the strength of the pathogenic factor involved. The thicker the coating, the stronger the pathogenic factor. Those factors which can be reflected in a thick coating are retention of food, dampness, phlegm, wind-cold or wind-heat, cold or damp-cold, and summer heat.

The thickness of the coating reflects only the strength of the pathogenic factor, not whether it is internal or external. Moreover, this rule applies only to thick coatings with root. If the coating is without root, its clinical significance is different. (See the discussion of coatings with and without root above.)

A thin coating indicates that the pathogenic factor is weak and that the disease is in its initial stage. However, a thin white coating is also normal and it is often impossible to determine whether or not such a coating is pathological. In this case, the practitioner must consider other factors, such as the distribution of the coating or the pulse. This is true, for example, in the early stages of invasion by wind-cold where the coating is thin, reflecting the weak nature of the pathogenic factor. Analysis of the thickness and color of the coating alone is not useful here. One must observe the distribution of the coating, which, in the initial stages of an external attack, may be in the front third or around the central surface of the tongue. (Coating distribution and its clinical significance is discussed at greater length below.)

If the coating thickness reflects the strength of the pathogenic factor, it follows that any changes in the strength of the factor will be reflected by changes in the coating thickness. This fact is extremely useful in clinical practice for gauging the progress of a condition and establishing an accurate prognosis.

The significance of the thickness of the tongue coating is reflected in the following passage from the *Guide to Tongue Differentiation:*

If the tongue coating is dirty and thin, it means that the body's qi is weak; if it is dirty and thick, it means that the pathogenic factor is strong. If the coating is thin, the pathogenic factor is just beginning to manifest; if the coating is thick, the pathogenic factor is deep inside.[4]

Thus, if the coating becomes thinner it indicates that the body's qi is recovering or that the pathogenic factor is being expelled. If the coating becomes thicker it is a sign that the pathogenic factor is becoming stronger.

When a thick coating is present, treatment should be directed at expelling the pathogenic factor, whatever it may be. If herbs are used, prescriptions should be chosen which expel the particular pathogenic factor. If treatment involves acupuncture, the draining (also known as dispersing or reducing) method should be used.

If the tongue coating changes from thin to thick it indicates that the pathogenic factor is getting stronger and may be penetrating into the interior. In an acute, externally-contracted disease it is quite common for the change from thin to thick to occur rather quickly, in a day or even a few hours. In a chronic disease the change from thin to thick usually occurs more slowly, over the course of weeks. If, however, in the course of a chronic disease the coating suddenly changes from thin to thick, it indicates a serious weakening of the body's energies and the penetration of the pathogenic factor deeper into the interior. In this case, treatment should be directed at expelling the pathogenic factor while supporting the body's qi, in contrast to most cases in which a thick coating calls for simply expelling the pathogenic factor.

Generally speaking, a change in the coating from thick to thin indicates a positive development in the course of the disease, with a diminishment in the pathogenic factor's intensity. If, however, the coating suddenly changes from thick to thin, it reflects the sudden collapse of Stomach qi, whether in the course of an acute or chronic disease. This is always a bad sign and points to a poor prognosis. Treatment should aim at restoring and "rescuing" the Stomach qi quickly and vigorously.

It is important to distinguish between cases in which the thinning of the coating is due to an improvement of the condition and a diminishment of the pathogenic factor ("true thinning"), and cases in which the thinning of the coating actually points to a worsening of the condition ("false thinning").

In a true thinning the tongue coating changes from thick to thin, from stiff to soft and from dense to sparse. The thinning takes place from tip to root and a new, thin white coating appears underneath. All of these signs signify that the pathogenic factor has been expelled from the body and that the Stomach qi has been restored.

There are several varieties of false thinning apart from a sudden change of coating from thick to thin. All represent the worsening of a condition. When the coating disappears, no new coating is formed and the tongue is peeled and resembles a mirror, it indicates a collapse of Stomach qi. When the coating peels off but leaves patches looking like beancurd or cottage cheese scattered on the tongue, it indicates the collapse of Stomach qi and the exhaustion of Stomach fluids. When the whole tongue has a thick coating which disappears, leaving the tongue greasy or displaying red spots, another type of false thinning has occurred; within one or two days a new thick coating will be formed. Finally, when a thick coating disappears and the tongue surface is left shiny and dry, it signifies the exhaustion of Stomach qi.

Coating Distribution

The distribution of the coating over the surface of the tongue has a different clinical significance in conditions of externally-contracted versus internally-generated disease.

In externally-contracted disease the distribution of the coating is indicative of the location and depth of the pathogenic factor. In the initial stages of an externally-contracted disease the coating will be more concentrated either on the outside (around the central surface) or on the front part of the tongue. Furthermore, the change in distribution of the coating is an important sign of the advance or retreat of the pathogenic factor. For example, if a coating first appears on the front part or on the outside of the tongue (indicating a pathogenic factor's invasion of the exterior

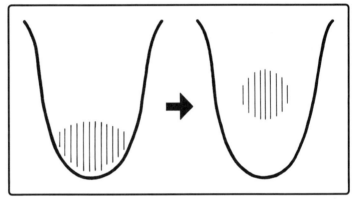

Illustration 7-3a

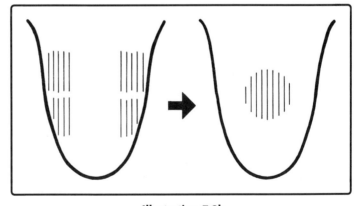

Illustration 7-3b

levels) and subsequently moves to the center, possibly also changing in color from white to yellow, then the pathogenic factor has penetrated to the interior. In this case, the initial coating on the front part or the outside of the tongue will not disappear. It will remain, but the coating on the tongue's central surface will become thicker (ILLUSTRATIONS 7-3a & b).

In cases of acute, externally-contracted disease, these changes in distribution take place in the course of a single day or even a few hours. If the patient is not examined every day or perhaps even twice a day from the inception of the disease onward, it will be difficult at best to draw conclusions from the changes in tongue coating distribution.

With respect to internally-generated diseases the distribution of the coating is not indicative of the progress of the pathogenic factor, but reflects the location of the problem in accordance with the norms of correspondence in tongue topography (see chapter 3).

In cases of internally-generated disease, one refers to *complete coating* (covering the entire tongue) or *partial coating* (covering only part of the tongue). The partial coating can be uneven in its distribution across the tongue's surface. A coating on the left side of the tongue alone indicates that the disease is in the Organs, and specifically the Liver. Usually, the left-side coating will also be rather slippery. A coating on only the right side of the tongue indicates that the disease is half-exterior and half-interior, i.e., a sign of the lesser yang pattern. Usually, this coating will be white and slippery. If, however, the coating on only the right side of the tongue is also thick, yellow and slippery, it may indicate retention of damp-heat in the Gallbladder, rather than the lesser yang pattern. The difference lies in the color of the coating.

A thin and slightly watery coating just behind the tip in the area corresponding to the Lungs indicates the retention of cold in the Lungs as a consequence of a prior and improperly treated attack of wind-cold.

Apart from those situations just described, the clinical significance of partial coating distribution should be viewed in relation to the areas of the tongue's topography which correspond to the Organs. For example, a thick coating on the central surface of the tongue indicates retention of food in the Stomach. If it is also slippery, it indicates retention of dampness in the Stomach. A thick coating on the root indicates retention of food in the Intestines. If it is also slippery and yellow, it indicates retention of damp-heat in the Bladder and/or the Intestines. In women, this area also corresponds to the Womb. A yellow, thick and slippery coating on the root can therefore also signify an infection in one of the pelvic organs.

Coating Moisture

A normal tongue coating will be slightly moist, indicating good supply and movement of the body fluids. Coating moisture provides an indication of the state of those fluids. If the coating is dry, it indicates that the fluids are insufficient, either from excess heat or yin deficiency. If the coating is too moist, it indicates excessive fluids or stagnation of fluids, either from external cold or internal cold from yang deficiency.

DRY COATING

A dry coating may appear for a variety of reasons. If the cause is excess heat in the Stomach, Lungs or Liver, the coating will be yellow; if from external wind-heat, the coating will be yellow and thin; if from Kidney yin deficiency, the tongue will be peeled, without coating; and if the cause is Stomach yin deficiency, the tongue will have a coating without root.

A special type of dry coating can arise from yang deficiency with retention of dampness. In this case the tongue will usually be excessively moist because the yang qi has failed to move the fluids, which then accumulate. But in severe cases of yang deficiency with retention of dampness, the dampness obstructs the qi. The qi is then unable to move and transform the fluids, and the deficient yang qi is also unable to move the fluids upward. As a result, the tongue becomes dry. In this case the mouth is dry, but there is no thirst; or, if there is thirst, the patient prefers to drink warm water in small sips. The absence of thirst is the critical symptom which differentiates this case from one of excess heat or deficiency heat, each of which can also cause a dry mouth.

WET COATING

A wet coating may also arise from a variety of causes. If the cause is yang deficiency with retention of dampness, the coating will be white. If the cause is exterior wind-cold, the coating will be white and thin.

There is an unusual type of wet coating that is caused by yin deficiency, a condition in which one would expect the coating to be dry (since fluids belong to yin). In this case, however, externally-contracted heat quickly penetrates to the blood level and causes the yin fluids to evaporate and flow upward to the tongue, causing a wet coating. This is, however, rather rare.

A special type of wet coating is the slippery coating. A slippery coating is excessively wet and has an oily appearance. It is rather sticky and is semitransparent. A slippery coating signifies that the yang deficiency is more severe than if the coating were less wet, and also that the deficiency of yang has led to the accumulation of fluids to the point of dampness or phlegm. This type of coating is described in *Guide to Tongue Differentiation:*

> A slippery coating indicates damp-cold, either from external or internal origin. If the pathogenic factor is only beginning to go inside, the tongue will have a white, slippery coating. . . If the coating is slippery and greasy, it indicates retention of damp-phlegm. If it is slippery, greasy and thick, it indicates retention of damp-phlegm and cold.[5]

Moldy or Greasy Coatings

It is important to distinguish the moldy from the greasy coating. The moldy (also called "rotten") tongue coating is rather thick and patchy, looks crumbly like beancurd (or cottage cheese) and can be scraped off the tongue, indicating that it is also without root. The clinical significance of the moldy coating is that it reflects the presence of heat in the Stomach. The heat transforms the dirty fluids (turbidity) of the Stomach and causes them to rise to the tongue. This condition is usually associated with yin deficiency of the Stomach, which creates more heat and renders the coating rootless. The coating is also yellow because of the heat. In clinical practice, moldy coating is often found in conjunction with abscesses and pus in the body.

The seriousness of a moldy coating is reflected in a passage from *Medical Sources:* "When Stomach and Kidney yin are deficient, damp-heat accumulates, moldy dampness evaporates upward and the tongue coating becomes moldy. This is always difficult to treat."[6]

Moldy coatings are often present in diseases diagnosed as serious from a biomedical perspective. The coating is often white and moldy when there is a lung abscess. Gastric ulcers often present with a yellow and moldy coating. In hepatitis, the coating is often gray and moldy, and the tongue body is purple.

Sometimes, a moldy tongue coating will also have white spots the size of rice grains. These indicate the transformation of the Stomach fluids into moldy turbidity.

A greasy tongue coating is thicker on the central surface of the tongue than it is on the edges. It is slippery but appears rougher than a slippery coating. It cannot be wiped or scraped off. The whole surface of the tongue is covered with a layer of sticky fluid, which has root and adheres firmly. There appear to be very many papillae and the surface of the tongue has a pronounced rough appearance.

A greasy coating indicates that the qi cannot transform the fluids, which then accumulate to form dampness or phlegm. A greasy coating is therefore frequently observed in cases of dampness or phlegm in their various manifestations, such as phlegm-heat, damp-phlegm,damp-heat or damp-cold. In each of these cases the tongue coating will be white or yellow, depending on whether there is cold or heat.

In clinical practice, there is not much difference between slippery and greasy coatings. The primary difference in appearance is that a slippery coating is really oily and shinier, and the papillae cannot be seen, while a greasy coating is rougher, more sticky than oily, not shiny, and the papillae seem greatly increased in number. The clinical significance of a slippery coating is that there is more retention of dampness, while a greasy coating indicates retention of phlegm. However, this distinction is by no means absolute, and both slippery and greasy coatings may indicate the presence of either phlegm or dampness.

The main difference in the clinical significance of a moldy versus a greasy coating is that the former indicates excess heat, while the latter is usually caused by yang deficiency. A moldy coating is also without root, indicating Stomach yin deficiency, while a greasy coating has root.

TONGUE COATING COLOR

Analysis of the tongue coating proper serves primarily to identify the depth and location of the pathogenic factor and the strength and integrity of the body's energies. In terms of the eight principles identification of patterns, analysis of the tongue coating proper is particularly useful in differentiating interior from exterior, and deficiency from excessive conditions. Analysis of the coating color, on the other hand, is more useful in differentiating hot from cold conditions in a very direct and simple way. This is the primary significance of the coating color in clinical practice. In addition, in the course of an acute illness the coating color also reflects the transformation of an exterior to an interior disease.

The coating reflects the state of the yang Organs more than that of the yin Organs, and its color accurately reflects the hot or cold nature of the condition. It follows that analysis of the coating color is of secondary importance in diagnosing diseases of the yin Organs, for which analysis of the tongue body color is of greater importance.

In acute conditions examination of the coating and its color is of primary importance. In chronic conditions it is more important to observe the tongue body color. This is because the tongue coating is more readily affected by short-term factors which do not affect the tongue body color as quickly. For example, a person may have had a pale tongue for many years due to yang deficiency. This person may develop a thick yellow tongue coating following the ingestion of spoiled food, with associated symptoms of loose, fetid-smelling stool, abdominal pain and a slight fever. In this case the acute condition caused by the temporary upset from spoiled food is reflected by a thick, yellow tongue coating which, in theory, is in contradiction to the pale tongue body color. This is only an apparent contradiction, however. The pale body color reflects the chronic condition, while the coating reflects a coexisting acute condition.

Analysis of the tongue coating color can provide an indication of the progress of a disease if changes in the coating can be regularly observed. A change of coating color from white to yellow generally reflects a transformation of the condition from cold to hot. It can also be regarded as indicating a progression from exterior to interior. A further change from yellow to gray and then to black is an indication of the pathogenic factor's continuing progress to the deeper levels. A change of color in the opposite direction, from black to gray to yellow to white, indicates an improvement in the condition and a diminishment of the pathogenic factor. This progression is described in *Guide to Tongue Differentiation:*

> When external pathogenic factors attack the body, the Organs lose their internal harmony and this is reflected on the tongue coating. If the tongue coating is white, the disease is in the exterior; if the tongue coating is yellow, the disease is in the interior; if it is gray-black, the disease is in the Kidneys. If the coating changes from white to yellow to gray to black, the disease is progressing; if the coating changes in the reverse order, health is returning.[7]

The color of the tongue coating accurately reflects not only the hot or cold nature of the condition, but also its interior or exterior characteristics and the degree of penetration of the disease. However, this sign alone should never be regarded as definitive. The tongue does not have a yellow or gray-black coating in every deep disease of the interior. Some of these conditions generate a thick white coating, which simply means that the disease is in the interior but has a cold nature. If in a deep disease of the interior the coating were yellow or gray-black, it would indicate that the interior disease is one of heat. Although it always reflects the hot or cold nature of a condition, the coating color can only be useful to gauge the degree of penetration of a pathogenic factor when its changes can be observed regularly over the course of the disease.

The four tongue coating colors discussed here are white, yellow, gray and black. These are the colors whose significance is generally recognized in China. Even though a brown coating is frequently seen in clinical practice, it will not be discussed separately because a brown tongue coating has the same clinical significance as a yellow one.

White Coating

A slightly moist, thin and white tongue coating is normal. When analyzing a white coating, one must first observe its thickness and moisture. A white coating is pathological if it is too thick, too thin, too wet or too dry. In certain conditions, the pathological coating is thin and white and only slightly too wet, in which case it is virtually indistinguishable from a normal coating. Such is the case in the initial stage of externally-contracted wind-cold, when the coating is thin (because the pathogenic factor is in the exterior and is just starting), white (because of the cold) and slightly moist (because the cold obstructs the movement of fluids).

Generally speaking, the white coating has three primary clinical meanings:

• *Cold.* First of all, with a few rare exceptions, a white coating indicates a cold pattern. Whatever the condition, if the coating is white it is generally caused by cold, which can be deficiency cold or excess cold, and either interior or exterior, depending on other signs. (There are rare cases in which a white coating is due to heat; nothing is absolute in Chinese medicine!)

• *Exterior.* In cases of externally-contracted disease, a white coating indicates the presence of an exterior condition. When such disease is acute, a white coating indicates that the pathogenic factor is still in the exterior and has not yet penetrated to the interior. If it does penetrate, it will appear as a yellow coating. A white coating can occur in some interior conditions that are not externally-contracted, in which case its interpretation is different.

• *Lung/Large Intestine Disease.* A white coating also reflects disease of the Lung and Large Intestine. A white coating on a stiff tongue body signifies an excess condition of the Lungs and Large Intestine. A white coating on a tender and flaccid tongue body indicates a deficiency condition of these Organs. If the coating is white and dry it may indicate dryness of the Large Intestine with hyperactivity of fire, or Lung yin deficiency with heat. Examination of the white coating alone is insufficient in forming these diagnoses. Other clinical signs must also be taken into account.

WHITE AND THIN

A uniformly thin, white and slightly moist coating is normal. In external attacks of wind-cold, wind-dampness or damp-cold the coating can also be thin, white and slightly moist. This type of coating is therefore not of particular clinical significance apart from indicating the presence of a cold pattern, if there is any disorder at all. This view is reflected in *A Compilation Regarding the Discussion of Cold-induced Disorders:* "In external attacks of cold, the coating shows no change; if the pathogenic factor of heat penetrates inward, the coating turns yellow."[8] In the context of externally-contracted diseases only, a thin, white tongue coating indicates that the pathogenic factor has not yet penetrated deeply.

WHITE, THIN AND SLIPPERY

This tongue coating is sometimes described as looking like rice soup. It is caused by an external attack of cold and dampness. A slippery and oily coating definitely indicates the predominance of dampness at the defensive qi level (of the four levels identification of patterns), which interferes with the Stomach and Lungs. Since these Organs cannot disperse fluids, a slippery coating results. As one Chinese medical text explains, "Defensive qi goes to the Stomach and Lungs when the external pathogenic factor attacks the exterior; if the tongue coating is white, the Stomach fluids cannot be transformed and the pathogenic cold turns into dampness."[9]

WHITE, THICK AND SLIPPERY

This tongue coating usually indicates an interior condition of dampness or cold with retention of food in the Stomach. The white color not only suggests the presence of cold, but also that the condition is not of very long duration. (If it were, the coating would be yellow or dirty gray.) It may also be the consequence of an external attack of cold, which has transformed into internal dampness.

WHITE, THIN AND DRY

This coating can result from several interior or exterior conditions. In interior conditions a thin, white, dry coating can be caused by deficient blood, in which case the tongue body will be pale. It can also be caused by yang deficiency when the yang qi is so deficient that it cannot move fluids; the coating therefore becomes dry. Note that the coating will normally be wet in a condition of yang deficiency.

In exterior conditions a white, thin and dry coating indicates that the Lung fluids have been injured by an attack of wind-cold or wind-heat and that the pathogenic factor is still in the exterior. In this case there will be fever and aversion to cold. If there is fever but no aversion to cold, it indicates that the external pathogenic factor has been cleared, but that the Lung fluids have been injured. It is easy to determine whether a dry coating is due to an external attack from a pathogenic factor or to internal heat: in the latter case, there will be thirst. When there is an exterior pathogenic factor and the coating is dry, one should not induce sweating (which would be the normal regimen for exterior attacks) because the Lung fluids are already injured.

A thin, white and dry coating can also indicate an external attack of dryness. As you would expect, this condition occurs primarily in hot and dry climates.

WHITE, THICK AND WET

This coating is found in external attacks from wind-cold when the pathogenic factor is strong (as reflected in the thickness of the coating). It can occur in greater yang or lesser yang patterns. In an internal condition a white, thick and wet coating indicates retention of damp-cold in the interior, usually in the middle burner.

WHITE, THICK AND DRY

This coating is usually found in interior conditions and is due to retention of turbid fluids inside with heat. This is one of the few cases in which a white coating signifies heat.

WHITE, THICK AND GREASY

This tongue coating is found in interior diseases and indicates yang deficiency of the Stomach and Spleen leading to retention of food or dampness. The coating is usually thicker in the center and root.

WHITE, THICK AND GREASY/SLIPPERY

This coating is very similar to the previous one except that it is more slippery and looks smoother and more oily. Also found in interior conditions, it indicates Spleen yang deficiency with retention of cold-damp-phlegm. It is sometimes described as looking like beancurd or, to use a Western analogy, like porridge or cottage cheese.

WHITE, THICK AND GREASY/DRY

Although it may seem contradictory for a coating to be both greasy and dry, this type of tongue coating is actually rather common in clinical practice. The term greasy here means that the coating has a rough, sticky appearance. It can either be on the wet, slippery side (in which case it is described as greasy/slippery) or on the dry side (in which case it is described as greasy/dry).

A greasy/dry coating signifies one of two possible conditions. First, the middle qi and the Stomach fluids may be deficient. The deficiency of the middle qi leads to the formation of phlegm. At the same time, the Stomach fluids are exhausted, making the coating dry. The second possibility is that there is internal heat with phlegm. In this case the heat makes the coating dry and the phlegm makes it greasy.

WHITE, ROUGH AND CRACKED

This type of coating is seen only in externally-contracted diseases. It is often encountered in attacks of summer heat, which injures the qi and gives rise to heat at the qi level (of the four levels differentiation). The coating is cracked from the heat but not dry because the heat is still in the qi stage, i.e., still rather superficial. This condition is found primarily in hot climates.

WHITE, STICKY AND GREASY

This type of coating, with bits of sticky fluid adhering to it, is due to dampness or phlegm from Spleen qi or Spleen yang deficiency. It is also found in attacks of dampness at the qi level in the course of an externally-contracted disease.

WHITE AND POWDER-LIKE

This coating resembles powder sprinkled on top of the tongue (PLATE 23). It is associated with several conditions including seasonal epidemic exterior heat, toxin in the interior, or externally-contracted heat in the Triple Burner.

WHITE AND SNOW-LIKE

This type of coating has white flakes, resembling snow flakes, scattered over the surface of the tongue. It signifies Spleen yang exhaustion (more severe than Spleen yang deficiency) with stagnation of damp-cold in the middle burner. The older Chinese medical texts call this condition "obstructed Spleen" to indicate the complete exhaustion of Spleen yang and its inability to resolve dampness.

WHITE AND MOLDY

This tongue coating has a sticky fluid adhering to it and is grayish-white in color. The scattered pieces of coating look moldy, somewhat like curdled milk (PLATE 5). This coating signifies Kidney and Stomach yin deficiency leading to heat, with damp-toxin lurking inside. This type of coating is only found in chronic conditions of long duration.

The origin of this coating is that deficient Kidney and Stomach yin are unable to transform the fluids, leading to the formation of dampness. The Stomach yin deficiency leads to a coating without root, resulting in the scattered appearance of the coating. The yin deficiency leads to deficiency heat. Long-standing retention of dampness, combined with the "steaming" from deficiency heat, causes the formation of a particularly obnoxious kind of dampness called damp-toxin. This expression means that the dampness has been retained for a long time and, combined with the deficiency heat, has fermented or become rotten. Textbooks often refer to this tongue as the "death tongue" to emphasize its serious implications. However, although it always represents a serious condition, it does not necessarily mean that death is imminent. Rather, it indicates that the body fluids have turned "moldy," and that the prognosis is poor.

HALF-WHITE AND SLIPPERY

This coating is generally white and thin on one side of the tongue, and white and slippery on the other. The two dissimilar halves of the coating are distributed vertically along the midline of the tongue. If the white, slippery coating is on the right side only, it indicates the lesser yang pattern (half-exterior, half/interior). If the white, slippery coating is on the left side only, it indicates a problem in the Organs, specifically in the Liver. This would confirm the view that the right side of the tongue reflects the condition of the Gallbladder (the lesser yang pattern being related to Gallbladder pathology), while the left side reflects the condition of the Liver. Another point of view holds that the right side corresponds to qi and the left side to blood. This is also consistent with what was said above. In the lesser yang pattern the pathogenic factor can be thought of as affecting the qi, and when the disease is in the Organs it affects the blood.

Yellow Coating

A yellow tongue coating has three broad meanings in clinical practice:

• *Heat.* A yellow coating gives an immediate and clear indication that the disease is of a hot nature, whether it is interior or exterior, deficient or excessive.

• *Interior.* In differentiating interior from exterior conditions, a yellow coating is generally interpreted to mean that the disease is in the interior. When a pathogenic factor first invades the body the tongue coating will be white; if it progresses inward to the interior, the coating will change from white to yellow. However, there are cases of external attack from wind-heat, summer heat or dryness when the pathogenic factor is still in the exterior but the coating is yellow. This is because the pathogenic factor itself is of a hot nature. Apart from such cases, if the patient is seen regularly during the course of a chronic condition and there are no exterior symptoms, it can be safely assumed that a yellow coating indicates that the disease is in the interior.

• *Stomach-Spleen Disease.* If the tongue coating is yellow it indicates Stomach and Spleen disease. If it is yellow and thick it indicates an excess condition of the Stomach and Spleen.

PALE YELLOW

A pale yellow coating is thin and white on the central surface, and pale yellow on the outside of the tongue. This signifies that the disease is about to turn from cold to hot, and from the exterior to the interior. "If the tongue coating is thin, light and yellow, it indicates heat in the Lungs which has not yet entered the Stomach."[10] A light yellow coating is frequently seen in external attacks of wind-heat, or wind-cold changing to heat. If the coating is light yellow but thick, it indicates the retention of dampness and heat in the middle burner, and stagnation of qi. This is frequently encountered in interior diseases.

YELLOW AND SLIPPERY

This tongue coating is frequently seen in clinical practice. It indicates the presence of damp-heat and may be found in cases of jaundice.

DIRTY YELLOW

This tongue coating is also caused by damp-heat, usually in the Stomach and Intestines. The dirty appearance indicates a long-standing retention of damp-heat.

YELLOW, STICKY AND GREASY

This tongue coating reflects the presence of heat and phlegm. If the yellow color is very dark and the coating very thick, it signifies great heat within the dampness such that the heat is primary and the dampness secondary. If the yellow color is light and the coating thin, it indicates great dampness within the heat such that the dampness is primary and the heat secondary.

DRY AND YELLOW

This coating reflects the presence of heat, which has injured the body fluids. This can occur with externally-contracted or internally-generated heat. In both cases, the presence of the coating in itself indicates that it is excess heat.

YELLOW ROOT WITH WHITE TIP

This coating started white and began to turn yellow as the external pathogenic factor penetrated deeper, turning into heat.

BILATERAL YELLOW STRIPS ON A WHITE COATING

The yellow strips occur on both sides of the tongue, while the remainder of the coating is white. In the course of an acute disease, this indicates that the external pathogenic factor is penetrating into the interior. In the course of a chronic internal disease, it indicates heat in the Stomach and Intestines.

THICK, BILATERAL YELLOW STRIPS AND YELLOW COATING

The two thick yellow strips of coating occur on both sides of the tongue (PLATE 4). This indicates heat in the Liver and Gallbladder. The thicker yellow strips of coating on the sides are also often slippery/greasy, which signifies the presence of dampness in addition to heat.

HALF-YELLOW, HALF-WHITE

A tongue longitudinally divided between yellow and white coatings indicates heat in the Liver and Gallbladder. More yellow on the right side corresponds to more heat in the Gallbladder, while more yellow on the left corresponds to more heat in the Liver.

Gray Coating

A gray tongue coating always signifies an interior condition and is found in conditions of both heat and cold. Whatever the clinical significance of a gray coating, it always means that the disease is of long duration. In other words, a gray coating develops from a yellow or white coating after a long time. There are only two basic types of gray coatings. A gray and dry coating is due to heat, while a gray and wet coating is due to cold.

GRAY, WET AND SLIPPERY

This coating indicates damp-cold in the Spleen. It usually evolves from a white coating.

GRAY AND DRY

This coating indicates a long-standing presence of heat, which has injured the body fluids. It usually evolves from a yellow coating, and generally means that there is heat from excess.

Black Coating

The clinical significance of a black coating is similar to that of a gray one. It can represent either a hot or cold pattern, and it always means that the disease is of long duration. A black coating evolves from a yellow or gray coating; black and dry indicates heat, and black and wet indicates cold.

BLACK, SLIPPERY AND GREASY

This coating covers the whole tongue and is rather thick. It signifies retention of damp-cold in the Stomach and Intestines.

BILATERAL BLACK STRIPS ON A WHITE COATING

In this case the coating is generally white except for thin, black strips on the sides of the tongue. It can mean that external cold has penetrated to the Stomach, which is deficient. The coating will also be wet. This interpretation is found in *Mirror of the Tongue in Cold-induced Disorders:* "This tongue coating shows that pathogenic factors of the greater yang and lesser yang stages have penetrated the Stomach. Therefore, the earth qi is extremely weak, which leads to icy cold limbs and a tight pain in the chest."[11] This type of coating may also reflect the presence of heat rather than cold, in which case it would be dry.

WHITE COATING, BLACK POINTS

When black points are scattered over the surface of a white coating which covers the tongue, it signifies the retention of heat in the interior following an attack by an external pathogenic factor. The white coating reflects the presence of an external factor while the black points signify that it has transformed into heat and has just penetrated the interior. With time the entire coating will become black.

WHITE COATING, BLACK PRICKLES

Prickles are fur-like projections protruding from the coating. It is considered a sign of true cold with false heat if the tongue is not dry, the prickles can be scraped away, the patient is thirsty but cannot drink, and the body feels hot. On the other hand, if the tongue coating is dry, the prickles are rough and can be felt pricking the hand and the patient feels hot, then a condition of pathogenic cold transformed into heat is indicated.

BLACK IN THE CENTER, WHITE AND SLIPPERY ON THE SIDES AND TIP

This coating indicates deficiency cold with dampness from Spleen yang deficiency.

HALF-WHITE AND SLIPPERY, HALF-YELLOW AND BLACK

In this case the tongue is longitudinally divided between a white, slippery coating on one side and a yellow and black coating on the other. If the left side is yellow and black, it signifies heat in the Liver. If the right side is yellow and black, it signifies heat in the Gallbladder.

YELLOW SIDES, BLACK AND GREASY CENTER

This coating indicates retention of damp-heat in the interior and is frequently observed in alcoholics. It signifies that heat has been retained in the Stomach. Stomach heat evaporates fluids, which condense and create Spleen dampness.

BLACK, DRY AND CRACKED

This coating reflects a severe, dangerous withering and exhaustion of the Kidney yin, the body fluids having been burnt out by heat. In rare and extreme cases this coating can also arise from true cold in the interior with yang deficiency, even though the tongue is dry. This happens when the yang qi cannot move and evaporate the fluids, which makes the coating dry. One should not mistake this for a heat pattern; it is really due to cold. The practitioner should look for other signs such as the absence of thirst and scanty, clear urine.

Multiple Coating Colors

In clinical practice the tongue coating frequently displays not one, but two or more different colors simultaneously. This is because in the course of a disease's pathological evolution the coating may only partially change color. Different parts of the tongue may display older or more recent coatings. This is often significant in following the progress of a disease. Sometimes the practitioner can gauge its past and future development by analyzing the different coating colorations on different parts of the tongue.

The following are examples of combinations of different colors that may occur on the same tongue coating.

WHITE AND YELLOW

When dealing with externally-contracted disorders, we have seen that white corresponds to the exterior and yellow to the interior. White also indicates cold, and yellow indicates heat. Thus, any coating which is partly white and partly yellow indicates that the condition is either just changing from an exterior to an interior one, or vice versa.

If the coating is mostly white with traces of yellow it means that the disease is an exterior one, but that it is about to change to an interior condition. If the coating is mostly yellow with traces of white, it indicates either that the disease has just changed from an exterior to an interior condition, or that it is just changing from an interior condition and that the interior heat is disappearing.

It is not possible to gauge exactly which way the disease is evolving unless the tongue can be examined daily. A further clue can be found in the location of the different coating colors. If the coating is white in the center and yellow around the center, it indicates that the pathogenic factor is just penetrating the interior and is transforming into heat. This factor should be considered in conjunction with other signs. If the patient still has aversion to cold, the pathogenic factor remains in the exterior.

If the coating is yellow in the center and white around the center, it indicates that the interior heat is starting to clear.

In chronic interior diseases, multiple coloration can frequently appear and be interpreted according to the location of the different coating colors. For example, white coating on the front part and yellow coating on the root of the tongue means that there may be an external attack of wind-cold coexisting with a condition of heat in the lower burner. Any other combination of white and yellow coating on different parts of the tongue can be analyzed in a similar way by referring to the tongue's topography of correspondences, and by recalling that white signifies cold and yellow signifies heat.

WHITE AND GRAY

If a coating with this combination is moist, it indicates the retention of damp-cold in the interior. If it is dirty, it indicates a long-standing retention of damp-cold-phlegm, with stagnation deriving from yang qi along with stagnation of yin qi. A coating that is half-white and half-gray, with either a vertical or horizontal division of the colors, signifies the retention of pathogenic cold in a half-exterior and half-interior state. This is the lesser yang stage of the six stages identification of patterns.

WHITE AND BLACK

A white coating with black points or a white, greasy coating with streaks of black indicates dampness in the Spleen at the qi level.

YELLOW AND BLACK

A tongue coating that is yellow in the center and slippery, greasy and black around the center means that there is damp-heat in the Spleen. This is an interior pattern.

If the coating is yellow on the sides of the tongue with black prickles on the central surface, it indicates heat in the yang brightness stage with desiccated stool in the bowels. This is the yang brightness Organ stage of the six stages identification of patterns.

WHITE, GRAY AND BLACK

A white coating on the central surface of the tongue with gray-black, greasy and slippery coating around it denotes retention of dampness in the Spleen.

YELLOW AND GRAY

In a constipated patient, a tongue coating that is dry and yellow in the center, and gray around the center, indicates that internal dampness has transformed into heat, which has injured the body fluids.

SUMMARY

The tongue coating is produced by the physiological digestive activity of the Stomach. A thin, white coating is normal. The main points to remember about the clinical significance of the tongue coating can be summarized as follows:

- Clinically, the tongue coating reflects the health of the yang organs, in particular the Stomach.
- The tongue coating, in contrast to body color and shape, can change quickly in color, thickness and distribution either as a result of treatment or pathological processes.
- The tongue coating can give an immediate and clear indication of the deficient or excessive character of a condition: the absence of coating always indicates deficiency, and a thick coating always indicates excess.
- In externally-contracted diseases, particularly in their initial stages, the coating assumes primary importance. In internally-generated chronic diseases the coating is of secondary importance relative to tongue body color and shape.
- The moisture and consistency of the coating is an important element in diagnosing the presence of phlegm or dampness: a slippery, greasy or sticky coating always indicates the presence of phlegm or dampness.
- The coating provides a clear indication of the hot or cold nature of a condition: white signifies cold, and yellow signifies heat. (Bear in mind that in a few cases these signs may contradict indications arising from the body color, e.g., a yellow coating on a pale body.)

NOTES

1. Zhang Xu-Gu, *Interpretation of the Discussion of Cold-induced Disorders (Shang han lun ben zhi)* (1835). Cited in Beijing College of Traditional Chinese Medicine, *Tongue Diagnosis in Chinese Medicine (Zhong yi she zhen)* (Beijing: People's Medical Publishing House, 1976), p. 39.

2. Zhou Xue-Hai, *Simple Study of Diagnosis from Body Forms and Facial Color.* Cited in *Tongue Diagnosis in Chinese Medicine,* p. 39.

3. D.W. Beaven and S.E. Brooks, *A Colour Atlas of the Tongue in Clinical Diagnosis* (London: Wolfe Medical Publications, 1988), p. 117.

4. Cao Bing-Zhang, A *Guide to Tongue Differentiation*. Cited in *Tongue Diagnosis in Chinese Medicine*, p. 40.

5. *A Guide to Tongue Differentiation*. Cited in *Tongue Diagnosis in Chinese Medicine*, p. 43.

6. Shi Shi-Nan, *Medical Sources*. Cited in *Tongue Diagnosis in Chinese Medicine*, p. 44.

7. *A Guide to Tongue Differentiation*. Cited in *Tongue Diagnosis in Chinese Medicine*, p. 46.

8. Zhang Lu, A *Compilation Regarding the Discussion of Cold-induced Disorders (Shang han jie lun)* (1667). Cited in *Tongue Diagnosis in Chinese Medicine*, p. 48.

9. *Interpretation of the Discussion of Cold-induced Disorders*. Cited in *Tongue Diagnosis in Chinese Medicine*, p. 49.

10. *Interpretation of the Discussion of Cold-induced Disorders*. Cited in *Tongue Diagnosis in Chinese Medicine*, p. 57.

11. Zhang Dan-Xian, *Mirror of the Tongue in Cold-induced Disorders*. Cited in *Tongue Diagnosis in Chinese Medicine*, p. 63.

TABLE OF TONGUE COATINGS

COATING COLOR	CLINICAL SIGNIFICANCE
White *or* white and thin	Wind, cold or dampness in the exterior (or normal)
White, thin and slippery	Exterior attack of damp-cold
White, thick and slippery	Dampness in the middle burner Cold with retention of food in the Stomach
White, thin and dry	Blood deficiency (body pale) Yang deficiency (body pale) Exterior attack of wind-cold or wind-heat, Lung fluids injured (body color normal) Exterior attack of dryness (body color normal)
White, thick and wet	Exterior attack of wind-cold (body color normal) Interior damp-cold in middle burner (body normal)
White, thick and dry	Dirty fluids in the interior with heat
White, thick and greasy	Yang deficiency with retention of food or dampness
White, thick, greasy and slippery	Spleen yang deficiency with damp-cold or phlegm
White, thick, greasy and dry	Dampness with exhaustion of body fluids or heat

COATING COLOR	CLINICAL SIGNIFICANCE
White, rough and cracked	Attack of summer heat injuring the qi (qi level)
White, sticky and greasy	Dampness or phlegm in the middle burner Exterior attack of dampness at the qi level
White like powder	Exterior heat (body slightly red on tip or sides) Interior toxin (body red or dark red) Heat in the Triple Burner (body red)
White like snow	Spleen yang exhaustion with damp-cold in the middle burner
White and moldy	Kidney and Stomach yin deficiency, Damp-toxin in the interior
Half-white and slippery	Right side: pathogenic factor half-exterior, half-interior Left side: Heat in the Liver
Yellow or pale yellow	Exterior attack of wind-heat Wind-cold turning to heat Damp-heat in the chest and middle burner
Yellow and slippery	Damp-heat
Dirty yellow	Damp-heat in the Stomach and Intestines
Yellow, sticky and greasy	Heat and phlegm
Dry yellow	Heat-injured fluids
Yellow root, white tip	Exterior pathogenic factor just changing into heat and penetrating to the interior
Bilateral yellow strips (remainder white)	Exterior pathogenic factor penetrating to the interior Heat in the Stomach and Intestines
Bilateral yellow strips (remainder yellow)	Heat in the Liver and Gallbladder
Half-yellow, half-white (longitudinally)	Heat in the Liver and Gallbladder
Gray *or* gray, wet and slippery	Damp-cold in the Spleen
Gray and dry	Heat from excess
Black *or* black, slippery and greasy	Damp-cold in the Stomach and Intestines

COATING COLOR	CLINICAL SIGNIFICANCE
Bilateral black on white	Cold from deficiency of middle burner (wet) Heat from excess in the Stomach and Spleen (dry)
White coating, black points	Exterior pathogenic factor penetrating to the interior and transforming into heat
White coating, black prickles	True cold, false heat Cold turned into heat
Black in the center, white and slippery on sides	Spleen yang deficiency with damp-cold in the interior
Half-white and slippery, half-yellow and black	Heat in Liver or Gallbladder
Yellow sides, black and greasy center	Damp-heat in the Spleen and Stomach
Black, dry and cracked	Exhaustion of Kidneys Yang deficiency with interior cold

White and yellow	White in center, yellow around: pathogenic
	    factor just penetrating the interior and
	    changing into heat
	Yellow in center, white around: interior heat
	    just starting to clear

White and gray	White, gray and moist: damp-cold in the interior
	White, gray and dirty: damp-cold or phlegm
	    of long standing
	Half-white, half-gray: cold half-exterior, half-
	    interior

White and black	Dampness in the Spleen

Yellow and black	Yellow in center, black, slippery and greasy
	    around: damp-heat in the Spleen
	Yellow on sides, black prickles in center: heat
	    in the yang brightness stage
	Yellow, dry and black in center to tip: heat in
	    the Stomach and Intestines

White, gray and black (white in center, gray and black around)	Dampness in the Spleen
Yellow and gray (yellow in center, gray around)	Damp-heat with heat-injured fluids

Having concluded our discussion of tongue body color, shape, coating and moisture it may now be useful to highlight some of the more common imbalances in these aspects that occur in different parts of the tongue. The primary imbalances are those between tip and root, and between left and right. These are best illustrated in the table below.

TABLE OF
IMBALANCES BETWEEN TIP AND ROOT AND
BETWEEN LEFT AND RIGHT SIDES

	TIP-ROOT	LEFT-RIGHT
BODY COLOR	Tip and root of different color: stagnation of qi or blood	Different color on left and right: stagnation of qi
BODY SHAPE	a) Whole tongue swollen, tip more so: long-term problem, imbalance between Heart and Kidneys b) Only tip swollen: overwork	Only one side swollen, with red points: ipsilateral malnourishment of channels
COATING		Yellow coating on one side only: a) Gallbladder heat affecting the Stomach b) ipsilateral phlegm in the chest
MOISTURE	Tip red & dry, root dirty & swollen: defective transformation of body fluids	One side wetter: movement of fluids in the chest; Lung qi problem

8

Tongue Diagnosis in the Clinic

CLINICAL ISSUES WITH TONGUE DIAGNOSIS

One of the most useful aspects of tongue diagnosis is that the tongue body color nearly always shows the true character of the disharmony. This is especially helpful in complex and contradictory conditions, some examples of which will be described below. Our discussion will be articulated in seven parts:

- The tongue body color always shows the true condition
- The tongue does not necessarily show the *whole* condition
- When the tongue takes precedence over the pulse and symptoms
- When not to follow the tongue
- The tongue used to exclude serious internal Organ problems
- Integration of tongue and pulse diagnosis
- The tongue in prognosis

Tongue Body Color Always Shows the True Condition

The color of the tongue body is the most important and reliable aspect of tongue diagnosis because it always shows the true condition. This is especially useful in those situations where there are confusing manifestations of heat and cold, and of deficiency and excess. Some examples will clarify the importance of this aspect of tongue diagnosis.

KIDNEY YIN AND KIDNEY YANG DEFICIENCY

When there is deficiency of both Kidney yin and yang (which is relatively common, especially in women) the clinical manifestations may be contradictory.

For example, a woman may suffer from backache, frequent and pale urination, cold feet, slight edema of the ankles (all signs and symptoms of Kidney yang deficiency), as well as night sweats (a symptom of Kidney yin deficiency). On the other hand, another woman may suffer both from night sweats, hot flushes, dry throat and eyes (all symptoms of Kidney yin deficiency), and from cold feet and pale urine (symptoms of Kidney yang deficiency). Both of these conditions are more likely to appear in women over forty. Unless the pulse is clearly floating and empty, signifying Kidney yin deficiency, or very deep and slow, denoting Kidney yang deficiency, it may not be of much help in differentiating between the two conditions. In fact, in both Kidney yin and Kidney yang deficiency the pulse may simply be weak at both proximal positions.

Thus, in such contradictory conditions, the color of the tongue body is vital in determining the true character of the disorder. If the tongue body color is pale, Kidney yang deficiency predominates, and if it is red, Kidney yin deficiency predominates. In the former case one should tonify and warm the Kidney yang, and in the latter nourish the Kidney yin. The importance and significance of the tongue body color is such that one can safely choose the treatment strategy based upon it.

The following brief case history serves to highlight this principle. A woman of 45 had been suffering from night sweats and severe hot flushes for several weeks. While these two symptoms pointed to yin deficiency, she also felt cold in general, her feet were cold, urination was frequent and pale, and, most of all, the body of her tongue was very pale. This indicated that she suffered from a deficiency of both Kidney yang and Kidney yin, with a predominance of the former.

Because of this, I adopted the treatment principle of tonifying and warming the Kidney yang and used direct moxibustion with seven moxa cones on CV-4 *(guan yuan)*. Although this technique would appear to have been contraindicated by her hot flushes, the results were excellent: the hot flushes which she had suffered for six weeks were stopped with just one treatment.

EMOTIONAL PROBLEMS

Where there are emotional disorders the tongue is a very reliable indicator of the true origin of the problem. Generally speaking, for long-standing emotional disorders either the whole tongue or only the tip becomes red. This is due to the fact that every emotional strain (whatever the type of emotion) upsets the normal rising and descending of qi, which over time will stagnate. Long-standing stagnation of qi, on the other hand, leads to heat or fire. Because the Heart houses the spirit, which is affected by all types of emotions, Heart heat or Heart fire will develop. And because the tongue is the offshoot of the Heart, and its tip specifically corresponds to the Heart, either the whole tongue or only its tip will become red. It is for this reason that a red tip to the tongue is such a common finding in long-standing emotional disorders (PLATES 8, 18 & 47).

However, although emotional problems are by far the most common cause of a red tip to the tongue, they are not the only cause. In a few cases the tip of the tongue may become red due to overwork. Barring this reason, which is fairly rare, a red tip to the tongue is therefore a very reliable indicator that the basis of disharmony is emotional in nature. Thus, in the course of examining a patient, it is essential to observe whether or not the tongue (or its tip) is red, and the extent of its redness.

A careful examination of the tongue, and its integration with the pulse, always provides reliable information about the origin of a disharmony. For example, a person may be very depressed, tired, move very slowly and speak in a decidedly low voice, all of which would suggest a condition of deficiency and the presence of such emotions as sadness or grief. However, if the tongue is dark red with redder sides and tip, this definitely indicates that anger rather than sadness is the cause of the depression. On the other hand, although a person may look restless and anxious, if the tongue is *not* red, or only slightly red on the tip, sadness or grief may be the real cause of the disharmony.

Let us take an example of a different situation: a person may look very anxious and be restless, but if the tongue is pale this indicates that the spirit is restless from a general deficiency of qi and blood, which in this case affects the spirit and causes an emotional disturbance, rather than the other way round.

The Heart crack described in chapter 6 is another reliable indicator in emotional problems. If a person is subject to considerable emotional stress with severe anxiety and mental restlessness and has a red tongue, the presence of a Heart crack (in the midline extending to just behind the tip) indicates that the patient has a constitutional tendency to a Heart pattern, and that the problem will therefore be more difficult to treat. If, however, the same manifestations appear with *no* Heart crack, the condition is not so deeply rooted and should be easier to treat.

SPLEEN YIN AND STOMACH YIN DEFICIENCY

Sometimes the tongue may show a certain condition very clearly even though other signs and symptoms are absent. In these cases the tongue signs are such clear evidence that they may be relied upon and the patient may be given preventive treatment. Two cases in point are Spleen yin or Stomach yin deficiency.

With Spleen yin deficiency the tongue has very distinct small transverse cracks on the sides (ILLUSTRATION 6-13 and PLATES 29 & 34) and is generally dry. This indicates long-standing deficiency of Spleen yin, the manifestations of which generally include those of Spleen qi deficiency plus a dry mouth, dry lips and dry stools. If the deficiency of Spleen yin is severe there may also be some symptoms of heat from deficiency, such as a feeling of heat in the face.

With Stomach yin deficiency the tongue also presents very clear and reliable signs: either a wide crack in the midline in the center of the tongue (ILLUSTRATION 6-14 & PLATE 25) or small scattered cracks (ILLUSTRATION 6-12 and PLATES 25 & 29). Occasionally the tongue may show such cracks even though there are no Stomach symptoms. In my experience such cracks are always diagnostic of a Stomach pattern which can be treated preventively before the appearance of symptoms.

The Tongue Does Not Necessarily
Show the Whole Condition

Although the tongue body color shows the true condition of the patient, it should be remembered that it does not necessarily show the *whole* condition. It needs to be integrated with other aspects of the disharmony, chiefly the pulse, complexion and symptoms. A patient's disharmony is a complex of various patterns, each of them manifesting more fully in a particular sphere of clinical manifestations. We therefore need to use tongue diagnosis dynamically in conjunction with other manifestations and not merely to confirm the diagnosis. A few examples will clarify this concept.

A woman may suffer from Liver blood deficiency leading to Liver yang rising, which causes headaches. Her tongue may be pale, reflecting the blood deficiency, and her pulse wiry, reflecting the rising of Liver yang. If she has other symptoms of Liver yang rising, such as a slightly red complexion and a dry throat, when we integrate these symptoms with the wiry pulse we may be baffled by the pale color of the tongue. In fact, most books will say that with Liver yang rising, the tongue (or its sides) will be red. However, if we understand the principle that the tongue may show only *a part* of the configuration of patterns, we realize that the tongue is reflecting the deficiency of Liver blood, and the pulse and symptoms the rising of Liver yang (ILLUSTRATION 8-1).

LIVER BLOOD DEFICIENCY ⎯⎯⎯⎯⎯⎯⟶ **LIVER YANG RISING**
(PALE TONGUE)   (WIRY PULSE, RED FACE, ETC.)

Illustration 8-1

The example of a tongue when there is a deficiency of both Kidney yin and Kidney yang has already been discussed above. In that case the tongue reflects only part of the configuration of patterns, i.e., the predominant deficiency (ILLUSTRATION 8-2).

KIDNEY YANG DEFICIENCY − − −AND− − −**KIDNEY YIN DEFICIENCY**
(PALE TONGUE, FEELING COLD)   (NIGHT SWEATS, ETC.)

Illustration 8-2

Another striking example of how the tongue may reflect only part of a condition occurs in skin diseases. In many cases of chronic skin disease there is wind-heat, damp-heat or heat in the blood (or a combination thereof) which causes the skin lesions to become very red, itchy and hot to the touch. With such striking manifestations of heat in the skin one would expect the tongue to be red. However, because there is often a background of blood deficiency in chronic skin diseases, the tongue is often pale. If we disregarded the principle that the tongue may show only one aspect of a configuration of patterns, we would again be baffled (ILLUSTRATION 8-3).

BLOOD DEFICIENT AND DRY ───────➤ HEAT IN THE BLOOD
(PALE TONGUE)   (RED-HOT-ITCHY SKIN LESIONS)

Illustration 8-3

Another very common case in which the tongue reflects only one aspect of a disorder is that of Spleen qi deficiency leading to dampness or phlegm. In women Spleen qi deficiency also frequently leads to blood deficiency and dryness. While one would therefore expect the tongue to be thin and dry, in fact it is nearly always found to be pale, swollen and with a sticky coating. This occurs because the tongue is reflecting the Spleen qi deficiency and dampness/phlegm, but not the blood deficiency (ILLUSTRATION 6-1).

Yet another case in which the tongue does not show the whole condition is when a certain pattern is "incorporated" within another. For example, Liver blood deficiency may evolve into Liver yin and/or Kidney yin deficiency after some years. The tongue would have been pale initially, and become red and peeled with the onset of Liver yin deficiency. Liver yin deficiency will, of course, manifest with its own characteristic signs and symptoms, but some of those associated with Liver blood deficiency may remain. In this case the tongue is unable to show both conditions because it obviously cannot be both pale (Liver blood deficiency) and red (Liver yin deficiency) at the same time. Here we say that Liver blood deficiency has been incorporated within Liver yin deficiency. We must therefore pay attention to the symptoms and nourish Liver blood as well as Liver yin.

When the Tongue Takes Precedence
Over the Pulse and Symptoms

In many instances the treatment strategy should be based on the appearance of the tongue rather than the symptoms. Some examples will clarify this concept.

Many patients will present with localized heat signs even though the underlying condition is characterized by yang deficiency or cold. Although it is imperative that the heat signs be treated, the underlying condition, as evidenced by the appearance of the tongue, must be the primary focus of treatment.

Consider the following case history. A 35-year-old woman had been suffering from inflammation and swelling of the left eye; the sclera was red and the eye always felt irritated. All of these symptoms clearly pointed to heat affecting the eye. Her tongue, however, was very pale and she had other signs and symptoms of Spleen yang deficiency. In modern China the tendency in such cases is to completely ignore the tongue and follow the symptoms. As a matter of fact, this patient (a practitioner of acupuncture) had been treated with Chinese herbs while studying in China. But not only had this failed entirely to help the eye, it had also made her worse in other ways, causing diarrhea and abdominal pain.

I examined one of the packets of herbs which she had brought back and noticed that the ingredients were all cold-bitter herbs to drain fire from the eyes. In treating this patient I followed the principle of giving precedence to the appearance of the tongue and treated the patient accordingly. I therefore prescribed a formula to tonify Spleen qi, adapted with the addition of a few herbs which gently clear heat from the eyes. This not only produced an improvement in her general condition, but also helped the eye.

An example of a contradiction between the tongue and symptoms has already been described above, in which the symptoms showed heat in the blood and the tongue showed blood deficiency and dryness. Although in such cases it is important to address the condition of heat in the blood, nourishing and moistening of the blood should not be overlooked.

Patients suffering from carcinoma of the lung may develop a fever followed by symptoms of dryness, such as a dry throat. Very often, however, the tongue is pale, tooth-marked and has a sticky coating, which are indications of Spleen qi deficiency and dampness. In this case one should not nourish the yin (in accordance with the symptoms) but tonify the Spleen qi and resolve dampness (in accordance with the appearance of the tongue).

When Not to Follow the Tongue

There are cases when one needs to base the treatment strategy on the symptoms rather than the tongue, at least initially. Heat and cold can coexist and there are cases when the symptoms show heat but the tongue shows cold. In most cases it is better to deal with the heat first and the cold later. This is especially desirable when heat and cold coexist in the same system, e.g., Bladder and Kidneys (see below).

A very common example would be that of a patient suffering from urinary problems from damp-heat in the Bladder, but with an underlying deficiency of Kidney yang. The former pattern would cause signs and symptoms of heat, such as burning on urination and dark urine, while the latter pattern will present with such symptoms as backache and feeling cold. This situation is common in women with urinary symptoms or men with prostate problems. In such cases, initially at least it is necessary to ignore the tongue and clear the damp-heat from the lower burner.

Another example is that of cases when all the signs and symptoms *except* the tongue point to a certain condition. It may be that the patient has reached a period of life, usually in the mid-forties, when the tongue is about to change color. For example, a woman of 44 may suffer from frequent and pale urination, edema of the ankles, a feeling of cold, diarrhea, backache, dizziness and tiredness, and her pulse may be very weak at both proximal positions: all of these signs and symptoms point clearly to Kidney yang deficiency, and the tongue should accordingly be very pale. If it is not, we are probably seeing the patient at that moment in time when the condition is just about to change from yang to yin deficiency. This example, taken from an actual case, illustrates the principle in diagnosis of "looking not only at the horizon, but also over the horizon," i.e., not regarding the clinical manifestations as static at a given point in time, but being aware of the time scale and how the condition is changing over time.

Tongue Used to Exclude Serious Internal Organ Problems

It is very important to check the appearance of the tongue in order to exclude or rule out the possibility of serious internal Organ disorders, especially when there are emotional problems. For example, if a person appears very tense, anxious and distraught and the pulse is wiry and rapid, one immediately checks these manifestations against the tongue: if the tongue is *not* red, the tongue body not abnormal and the coating not very thick, the emotional stress has not yet seriously affected the internal Organs. The problem is therefore still at the level of qi, rather than nutritive qi or blood. If, on the contrary, the tongue is dark-red, peeled and cracked, this definitely denotes that the internal Organs have been seriously affected by the emotional stress over a long period of time.

Another example relates to asthma. The tongue is one of the manifestations which allow us to distinguish between allergic and non-allergic asthma. In early-onset allergic asthma the tongue body is usually not swollen, while in nonallergic asthma, corresponding to the breathlessness disorder *(chuăn)*, it is usually quite swollen. This is because the former usually is not due to phlegm, while the latter is. Although in both types of asthma the internal Organs are affected, in the nonallergic, late-onset type the Lungs and Spleen are more seriously distressed by the presence of phlegm.

Integration of Tongue and Pulse Diagnosis

The integration of tongue and pulse diagnosis is extremely important in the diagnostic process. Tongue and pulse manifestations are usually perfectly complementary, and their integration leads to a more reliable diagnosis. The principles of integrating tongue and pulse diagnosis can be articulated under the following headings:

- Qi and blood
- Time factor
- When the pulse is rapid and the tongue is not red
- Degree of detail
- Emotional problems

QI AND BLOOD

The pulse and tongue are complementary because, generally speaking, the pulse reflects qi and the tongue reflects blood (as it is the offshoot of the Heart, which governs blood). Although this is not always true — the pulse can reflect the state of blood (e.g., a choppy pulse) and the tongue can reflect the state of qi — it is nevertheless a useful generalization. Observation of the tongue adds another dimension to the findings of the pulse, showing how severe, deep or long-standing the condition is, and whether or not it is affecting the blood.

For example, in some cases the pulse may be wiry and rapid due to emotional problems. Here examination of the tongue allows us to differentiate between a deep, long-standing emotional problem which has affected the blood (when the tongue is deep-red with a dark-yellow coating), and a less serious one which has affected only the qi (the tongue is not red, or is only slightly red on the tip).

TIME FACTOR

It is also useful to check the tongue against the pulse because the latter is more subject to short-term influences than is the tongue. The tongue is thus used to rule out certain conditions which may otherwise be indicated by the pulse. For example, the pulse may become rapid due to exercise or a short-term emotional upset, whereas the tongue will not change. As another example, the pulse may become quite weak from overwork after only a few weeks, whereas the tongue will not change in that span of time.

The tongue is also a useful indicator of the duration of a problem. For example, it generally takes a long time for the tongue to become purple; thus, if the tongue is purple we may assume that the problem began to develop at least several years before.

Finally, the tongue is helpful in giving us an idea of what *stage* a problem has reached, i.e., it allows us to "look over the horizon" and see both the origin of the problem in the past and how it is likely to develop in the future. A good example of this is the development of yin deficiency as reflected on the tongue coating (ILLUSTRATION 7-2).

WHEN THE PULSE IS RAPID AND THE TONGUE IS NOT RED

Apart from short-term emotional upsets, the pulse may also become rapid due to a shock that occurred many years before. The appearance of the tongue, being *not* red, may help to confirm that the pulse is rapid not because of heat, but because of shock. In addition, the left distal pulse would be slightly overflowing.

Another case in which a rapid pulse is not associated with heat is when a person with weak Heart qi overworks for a long period of time. This causes Heart qi deficiency, but because the person constantly pushes him- or herself, the qi tries to compensate and the pulse accordingly becomes rapid. Because this is not caused by heat the tongue will not be red, but may have a Heart crack flanked by a slight swelling on either side (PLATE 8). The pulse may also be slightly overflowing at the left distal position.

DEGREE OF DETAIL

The pulse may be a more exact instrument than the tongue in pinpointing the origin of a problem. For example, if the tongue root has a sticky-yellow coating with red spots, it indicates retention of damp-heat in the lower burner, but from the tongue alone we may be unable to distinguish whether this is in the Bladder, Intestines, or Womb. By integrating our findings from the tongue with those from the pulse we may be able to determine this. In fact, if the pulse is wiry at the left proximal position the problem is usually in the Bladder; if it is wiry at both proximal positions it is usually in the Intestines; and if it is wiry at the pulse felt by rolling the finger toward the elbow at the left proximal position, the problem is in the Womb.

Another example of the detail offered by the pulse is in relation to Heart patterns. As we have seen, a Heart crack (in the midline extending to just behind the tip) is indicative of a constitutional tendency to Heart patterns. It is, however, essential to determine by means of the pulse whether this tendency manifests itself only as a Heart pattern, or as a heart problem in a biomedical sense as well. If there is a Heart crack, with the tip of the tongue being red, and the Heart pulse is either weak or slightly overflowing, the problem is only one of a Heart pattern due to emotional problems. However, if the Heart pulse is distinctly slippery on its edges (felt by rolling the finger sideways at the Heart position) while the rest of the pulse positions are not slippery, this suggests the possibility of an actual heart problem in a biomedical sense.

Yet another example is when the tongue is generally purple, indicating stasis of blood. In such cases the tongue alone will not indicate which Organ is so affected. However, the pulse position associated with the affected Organ will be wiry, or more wiry than the rest of the pulse if that is generally wiry. This allows us to identify which Organ is involved.

On the other hand, there are a few cases in which the tongue may help pinpoint the origin of a problem better than the pulse. For example, a very common pulse is one that is weak and deep at both proximal positions; this is frequently the case in people over 40 with Kidney deficiency. However, because both left and right rear positions are equally weak and deep, the pulse does not reveal whether it is Kidney yin or Kidney yang deficiency. The tongue will make the matter plain: it will be pale in Kidney yang deficiency and red in Kidney yin deficiency.

EMOTIONAL PROBLEMS

Where there are emotional problems which affect the Heart and cause the left distal pulse position to be overflowing while the pulse rate is normal, it is useful to check these findings against the tongue. If only the tip of the tongue is red, the emotional problem is recent and not too deep. If the whole tongue is red and the tip redder, it indicates an older and deeper emotional problem. If the whole tongue is red, the tip redder and there is a Heart-type crack (in the midline extending to just behind the tip), it means that the emotional problem is older and deeper, and also that the person has a constitutional tendency to emotional stress from a weak Heart. (The last case will be the most difficult to treat.) Thus the color of the tongue can provide a useful indication of the severity and depth of an emotional problem.

On the other hand, when the tongue has a central Heart crack this finding should be checked against the pulse. If the tongue is not red and the pulse is weak at both Heart and Kidney positions (left distal and proximal), this indicates a constitutional weakness of the Heart, and not an emotional problem.

To estimate the duration of an emotional problem it is useful to integrate palpation of the pulse with observation of the eyes and tongue. The eyes readily reflect emotional problems for they become dull and lose their radiance. In comparative terms, when there is an emotional problem the pulse changes first, then the eyes and finally the tongue. The integration of these three aspects of diagnosis may thereby enable us to form a clearer idea of how long-standing and deep-rooted an emotional problem is.

The Tongue in Prognosis

The tongue is an excellent tool for making a prognosis in Chinese medicine. Prognosis often involves a quantitative assessment of the condition. While Chinese medicine stresses more the qualitative aspect, it does not ignore quantitative appraisal altogether. The tongue can play an important role in this process.

Five aspects of prognosis based on the tongue will be considered here:

- Strength of pathogenic factor
- Purple color
- Yin deficiency
- Surgical operations
- Bone fractures

STRENGTH OF PATHOGENIC FACTOR

First of all, because the thickness of the tongue coating has a direct relationship to the intensity of a pathogenic factor, it enables us to make a prognosis. Thus, e.g., if two people fall ill with an acute chest infection, the prognosis for the one with a thinner coating is better.

The coating also assists in prognosis when it appears or disappears suddenly. In fact, if a tongue without coating suddenly develops a thick one, or if a thick coating suddenly disappears, both are signs of a poor prognosis. This question is discussed more fully in chapter 7.

PURPLE COLOR

The tongue body color is also very important in prognosis, especially the color purple. Generally speaking, it takes a long time for a tongue to become purple; thus, this color usually indicates both that the condition is long-standing and that the prognosis is less promising than other tongue body colors.

A purple color on the sides of the tongue in the area between the tip and center indicates stasis of blood in the chest in general, or in the breasts in women (ILLUSTRATION 5-4). Specifically, in a woman with breast cancer the color purple in this area (which reflects an affliction of the ipsilateral breast) indicates a poor prognosis. The more purple it is, the worse the prognosis.

The color purple also indicates a poor prognosis when it appears in patients suffering from digestive symptoms of the stomach. An article in the *Journal of Traditional Chinese Medicine* reported the tongue signs which herald a poor prognosis in patients with gastric symptoms. These are primarily a purple color on the tongue body, purple spots or a purple color of the sublingual veins.[1]

YIN DEFICIENCY

The presence or absence of tongue coating is also a helpful factor in prognosis in cases of yin deficiency. A deficient yin tongue is usually described as red and completely without coating (peeled), but this represents an advanced stage of yin deficiency. The tongue progresses through various stages before reaching this point. As the progression to a red and completely peeled tongue follows fairly predictable stages, by analyzing the coating (or lack of it) we can identify the stage of the progression and therefore the prognosis.

In examining the tongue for yin deficiency one should pay particular attention to two aspects:

• *Coating:* an absence of coating or a rootless coating indicates yin deficiency.
• *Body color:* if the coating is missing and the body is red, it means that yin deficiency has given rise to deficiency heat.

It is important to realize that these two aspects are quite independent, i.e., yin deficiency does not automatically lead to deficiency heat. It is entirely possible to have yin deficiency without deficiency heat. This condition will manifest on the tongue with an absence of coating or with a rootless coating, while the body is *not* red (PLATE 25). Because the coating is formed by the digestive activity of the Stomach, yin deficiency always begins with Stomach qi deficiency.

As discussed in chapter 7, we can map the progression of a tongue to complete yin deficiency through the following stages (ILLUSTRATION 7-2):

1. Normal body color and a thin, white coating with root: the normal state.

2. Normal body color and a rootless coating in the center: the beginning of Stomach qi deficiency.

3. Normal body color and a rootless coating all over: a further progression of Stomach qi deficiency.

4. Normal body color, a rootless coating all over with peeling in the center: Stomach yin deficiency. If the center is also red this denotes that Stomach yin deficiency has given rise to deficiency heat in the Stomach only (PLATES 12 & 20).

5. Normal body color and coating entirely absent (completely peeled): a further stage of Stomach yin deficiency. In such cases there will typically be a Stomach crack (PLATE 25).

6. Red body color and a completely peeled tongue: Stomach and Kidney yin deficiency with the development of deficiency heat. In such cases there may be a central Stomach crack and other scattered cracks, a sign of more severe yin deficiency and consequent dryness (PLATES 13 & 24).

Obviously, this is only a theoretical progression of the development of yin deficiency. In practice there are variations in these stages.

SURGICAL OPERATIONS

The tongue body color usually becomes pale (or if already pale, paler) after surgical operations, especially those of the digestive system. Thus, if the tongue becomes red (or redder) after an operation, it indicates a poor prognosis, such as the development of complications.

BONE FRACTURES

A study of 122 patients with bone fractures showed that generally the tongue becomes purple or develops purple spots within one week of the occurrence of a bone fracture.[2] The time required for the purple color to disappear after the mending of the bones varies with the age of the patient, and is faster in young people. In fact, patients under 20 may not develop a purple tongue at all.

If the tongue becomes red and peeled after a bone fracture it indicates a poor prognosis. The patient may have pain in the affected limb and the bones may not mend well. In such cases the tongue becomes red and peeled from stagnant blood turning into heat and injuring yin.

TONGUE DIAGNOSIS AND HERBAL THERAPY

The appearance of the tongue not only provides a crucial guide to diagnosis but is also an essential indicator in herbal therapy. Three aspects of this concept will be considered here:

- Tonifying the body's qi versus eliminating pathogenic factors
- Differentiation of Stomach/Spleen, qi/yin deficiency
- Differentiation of heat at the qi or nutritive qi and blood level, and between heat and fire

Tonifying the Body's Qi Versus Eliminating Pathogenic Factors

The most fundamental choice of treatment strategy is that between tonifying the body's qi and eliminating pathogenic factors. This choice is more crucial with herbal medicine than with acupuncture because in herbal medicine there is a sharp distinction between a formula that primarily tonifies the body's qi (e.g.,

Four Gentlemen Decoction *[si jun zi tang]* to tonify qi) and one that primarily eliminates pathogenic factors (e.g., Agastache, Magnolia, Pinellia, and Poria Decoction *[huo po xia ling tang]* to resolve dampness).

The tongue is a very important indicator in choosing between tonifying the body's qi and eliminating pathogenic factors. If the tongue clearly shows that pathogenic factors are strong and predominant, then it is safe to concentrate one's attention on eliminating them. Aspects of the tongue which show a predominance of pathogenic factors include:

- A very thick coating indicates prevalence of dampness, phlegm, retention of food or other external pathogenic factors
- A very swollen tongue body denotes dampness or phlegm
- A very dark red body color indicates extreme heat or fire if the tongue has a coating, or deficiency heat if it has no coating
- A very stiff tongue body denotes the presence of internal wind

Let us take the example of two tongues, one which is pale, tooth-marked and with a thin, white coating, and the other of which is also pale, but is very swollen and has a sticky coating. The former indicates primarily Spleen qi deficiency and calls for tonification with a formula such as Four Gentlemen Decoction *(si jun zi tang)*. The latter also denotes Spleen qi deficiency, but the swelling of the tongue body and the sticky coating signify that dampness or phlegm are predominant; it might therefore be better to start with a formula that resolves dampness, such as Agastache, Magnolia, Pinellia, and Poria Decoction *(huo po xia ling tang)* in cases of damp-cold, or Coptis and Magnolia Decoction *(lian po yin)* in cases of damp-heat.

To give another example related to the tongue body color, we can take two tongues, one of which is slightly red and peeled, and the other very dark red, with a redder tip, and peeled. The former tongue denotes the presence of heat from yin deficiency, but since it is only slightly red, yin deficiency predominates; in treatment, attention can be directed at nourishing yin with no necessity of clearing the deficiency heat. The latter tongue, on the contrary, indicates the predominance of strong deficiency heat blazing upwards (because the tip is even redder); the treatment strategy here should therefore focus primarily on clearing the deficiency heat (although the yin, too, should obviously be nourished).

Differentiation of Stomach/Spleen, Qi/Yin Deficiency

The tongue can be extremely helpful in distinguishing between the conditions of Spleen qi deficiency, Stomach qi deficiency, Stomach yin deficiency and Spleen yin deficiency, and can point to the relevant herbal formulas. While the differentiation of these conditions may be difficult on the basis of symptoms and pulse alone, it becomes clear when the appearance of the tongue is taken into account (TABLE 8-1).

PATTERN	TONGUE	HERBAL FORMULA
Spleen qi deficiency	Slightly swollen or swollen sides, tooth-marked, sticky coating	Six-Gentlemen Decoction *(liu jun zi tang)*
Stomach qi deficiency	Rootless coating	Ginseng, Poria, and Atractylodes Macrocephala Powder *(shen ling bai zhu san)*
Stomach yin deficiency	No coating in the center, possible Stomach crack, dry	Glehnia and Ophipogonis Decoction *(sha shen mai men dong tang)*
Spleen yin deficiency	Rootless coating, transverse cracks on the sides, dry	Ginseng, Poria, and Atractylodes Macrocephala Powder *(shen ling bai zhu san)*

Table 8-1: Qi/Yin Deficiency Patterns and Herbal Formulas

Differentiation of Heat at the Qi or Nutritive Qi and Blood Levels, and between Heat and Fire

Another important application of tongue diagnosis to herbal therapy is in connection with heat disorders. Here it is essential to distinguish both between heat from excess versus that from deficiency, and, within the category of heat from excess, to distinguish between fire and heat. Since the relationship between red tongues and heat disorders is closely linked historically with the school of warm diseases, it will be useful to discuss this question from the perspective of the identification of patterns according to the four levels: defensive qi, qi, nutritive qi and blood (APPENDIX II).

While the first level describes the clinical manifestations induced by external wind-heat, the other three are concerned with the signs and symptoms of heat. However, there are important differences between the heat of the qi level and that of the nutritive qi and blood levels. Moreover, within the qi level itself there are crucial differences among the various patterns, some of which are patterns of heat and some of fire.

At the qi level one can distinguish patterns of heat from those of fire. Heat is nonsubstantial and floats toward the surface. Its main manifestations are a feeling of heat, body feeling hot to the touch, thirst, sweating and an overflowing pulse. Heat is in the Organs, but not yet at a deep level, and it has a tendency to push outwards: the overflowing pulse is an expression of this phenomenon. Examples of heat are the patterns of Lung heat and Stomach heat at the qi level within the four-level identification of patterns, and that of the yang-brightness channel pattern within the six-stage identification of patterns.

Fire at the qi level is more substantial than heat. It is stronger than heat and is knotted deep inside where it dries up more, and affects the spirit more, than does heat; it may also cause bleeding. In particular, fire accumulates in the Intestines and desiccates the feces, causing constipation or dry stools. Fire toxin is also a type of fire. Examples of fire are the patterns of Intestinal dry-heat within the four-level identification of patterns, and that of yang-brightness Organ pattern within the six-stage identification of patterns.

At the nutritive qi and blood levels the heat injures the yin, drying up the body fluids. It is useful to have in mind the various types of Heat in relation to the Qi, Nutritive Qi and Blood levels (ILLUSTRATION 8-4).

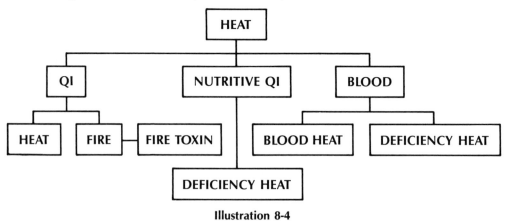

Illustration 8-4

The appearance of the tongue very clearly distinguishes among the types of heat involved (TABLE 8-2). Heat at the qi level manifests with a red body and a fairly thin yellow coating; it may even have only a yellow coating and a normal-colored body (PLATES 1, 33 & 36). Fire at the qi level has a more pronounced effect on the coating, making it very thick, dark yellow or brown (even black) and very dry. The tongue body will be red or dark red (PLATES 28 & 47). At the nutritive qi and blood levels the yin is injured and the tongue will definitely be red or dark red, and will *lack a coating,* i.e., will be peeled (PLATES 11,13, 24, 26 & 48).

The important point to note is that the above descriptions apply not only to acute, febrile diseases but also to any chronic, internal heat disorder. The appearance of the tongue provides a very clear and immediate clue as to what type of heat or fire is present. The distinction is important because the method of treatment varies greatly.

For qi-level heat one should adopt the method of clearing heat with pungent and cold herbs: cold to cool heat, and pungent to push the heat outwards toward the surface of the body. Examples of such herbs are Herba Lophatheri Gracilis *(dan zhu ye)*, Gypsum *(shi gao)*, Rhizoma Phragmitis Communis *(lu gen)*, Semen Sojae Praeparatum *(dan dou chi)*, Radix Bupleuri *(chai hu)*, Flos Lonicerae Japonicae *(jin yin hua)* and Rhizoma Anemarrhenae Asphodeloidis *(zhi mu)*. Examples

TYPE OF HEAT		TONGUE	TREATMENT PRINCIPLE
QI LEVEL	HEAT	Red or normal color, yellow coating	Clear heat with pungent-cold herbs
	FIRE	Red, thick, dry, dark-yellow, brown or black coating	Drain fire or move downwards
NUTRITIVE QI AND BLOOD LEVELS		Dark red, no coating, dry	Clear deficiency heat primarily, nourish yin secondarily

Table 8-2: Tongue Characteristics at Qi or Nutritive Qi and Blood Levels

of formulas that clear heat would include White Tiger Decoction *(bai hu tang)*, Lophaterus and Gypsum Decoction *(zhu ye shi gao tang)* and Drain the White Powder *(xie bai san)*.

For qi-level fire one should adopt the method of draining fire with bitter and cold herbs. These are often combined with the those that drain downwards, i.e., draining fire by purging. Examples of fire-draining herbs are Radix Gentianae Longdancao *(long dan cao)*, Radix Scutellariae Baicalensis *(huang qin)*, Rhizoma Coptidis *(huang lian)*, Cortex Phellodendri *(huang bai)*, Fructus Gardeniae Jasminoidis *(zhi zi)* and Radix Sophorae Flavescentis *(ku shen)*. An example of a formula that drains fire would be Gentiana Longdancao Decoction to Drain the Liver *(long dan xie gan tang)*. Herbs that drain fire by moving downwards include Radix et Rhizoma Rhei *(da huang)*, Mirabilitum *(mang xiao)* and Herba Aloes *(lu hui)*. Examples of downward-draining formulas are the three Order the Qi Decoctions *(cheng qi tang)* and Drain the Heart Decoction *(xie xin tang)*.

For nutritive-qi level heat one should follow the method of clearing heat primarily, and nourishing yin secondarily. Examples of herbs that clear deficiency heat at the nutritive-qi level are Rhizoma Anemarrhenae Asphodeloidis *(zhi mu)*, Herba Artemisiae Annuae *(qing hao)*, Herba Ecliptae Prostratae *(han lian cao)*, Rhizome Alismatis Orientalis *(ze xie)* and Cortex Lycii Radicis *(di gu pi)*. Examples of formulas that clear deficiency heat at the nutritive-qi level include Artemisia Annua and Soft-shelled Turtle Shell Decoction *(qing hao bie jia tang)*, Artemisia Annua and Soft-shelled Turtle Shell Powder *(qing hao bie jia san)*, Cool the Bones Powder *(qing gu san)* and Clear the Nutritive Level Decoction *(qing ying tang)*.

For blood-level heat one should clear deficiency heat and cool blood primarily, and nourish yin secondarily. If there is bleeding one should stop this by cooling the blood. Examples of herbs that clear deficiency heat and cool the blood are Cortex Moutan Radicis *(mu dan pi)*, Radix Rehmanniae Glutinosae *(sheng di huang)* and Radix Scrophulariae Ningpoensis *(xuan shen)*. Examples of formulas that clear deficiency heat and cool the blood include Guide Out the Red Powder *(dao chi san)*, Rhinoceros Horn and Rehmannia Decoction *(xi jiao di huang tang)* and Clear the Stomach Powder *(qing wei san)*.

TONGUE DIAGNOSIS IN CHILDREN

Tongue diagnosis in children presents certain differences from that of adults. The younger the child, the more differences there will be. After the age of seven or eight, a child's tongue presents few differences from that of an adult.

The first thing to note is that young children's tongues are naturally paler and wetter than those of adults. The younger the child, the paler and wetter the tongue. A survey of tongue features in 2721 normal Chinese children between the ages of 5 and 12 revealed that 166 had a wet or sticky coating.[3]

Children's tongues do not generally present many variations in tongue-body shape other than becoming swollen or thin. For example, yin-deficiency cracks are fairly rare in children.

Because children's tongues, unlike those of adults, are unencumbered by the accumulation of various pathological states over many years, they usually provide a very clear and immediate picture of the prevailing pathology.

Since invasion of external wind forms a major part of children's pathology, it is interesting to make some observation on the appearance of children's tongues during externally-contracted diseases. First of all, it should be noted that changes in body color subsequent to an invasion of external wind occur more frequently than in adults. Because children succumb much more readily to wind-heat than wind-cold, the tongue body color responds very quickly by becoming slightly red on the sides and/or front, signifying invasion of wind-heat on the exterior (ILLUSTRATIONS 4-1 & 4-2). Children also develop red points in such invasions much more readily than adults. The presence of red points on the sides and/or front indicates a greater intensity of the pathogenic factor. Thus, if a child suddenly develops a redness on the sides and/or front as well as red points, this is a very reliable indicator of an external invasion of wind-heat. In the absence of these signs, it may be that the child simply doesn't want to go to school!

It is important to note that redness and/or red points on the sides and/or front of the tongue actually appear *before* the onset of symptoms, and that these tongue signs are absolutely reliable. Thus, if one discovers these signs on the tongue, the child can be treated straightaway by expelling wind and releasing the exterior.

Likewise, if the tongue still shows pathological changes after the child seemingly improves, these signs are again absolutely reliable. In such cases it is important to continue treating on the basis of the tongue signs because children are very prone to develop residual pathogenic factors after external invasions. In fact, the presence of residual pathogenic factors, usually in the form of interior heat, phlegm-heat, dampness or damp-heat, is a major pathology in children accounting for a very large number of conditions such as repeated chest infections, wheezing, insomnia, recurrent ear infections, digestive problems, recurrent tonsillitis, swollen glands, etc. It is therefore of utmost importance to trust the tongue and continue treating after external invasions on the basis of these signs. In my practice whenever I treat a child for an acute respiratory infection due to invasion of wind-heat, I nearly always follow up the treatment after subsidence of symptoms with a formula to clear any residual heat, dampness or phlegm.

The signs showing the presence of a residual pathogenic factor depend on its character. In the case of Lung heat, the tongue may be red with red points in the front part, but extending toward the center. In the case of Lung phlegm-heat, the whole tongue will be red with a sticky yellow coating in the front extending toward the center. If dampness is the residual pathogenic factor, the tongue will have a sticky wet coating and may also have white vesicles.

Children are also prone to latent heat, which is clearly reflected on the tongue. Latent heat occurs when wind enters the body without causing immediate symptoms and penetrates into the interior, incubating for some weeks or months. After some time the latent heat emerges toward the surface, usually in conjunction with a new invasion of wind. The crucial difference from a normal invasion of wind-heat is that the child will have symptoms of interior heat *from the beginning,* i.e., irritability, insomnia, feeling of heat, thirst, weariness, etc. Most of all, the tongue will show signs of interior rather than exterior heat. It will be red or even dark red all over, and may also be partially peeled, i.e., it shows signs of interior heat at the nutritive-qi level. In such cases, it is important that attention be directed at clearing interior heat from the beginning, rather than expelling wind and releasing the exterior.

Another characteristic of children's tongues during acute invasions of external wind is that the appearance of the tongue can change very quickly, sometimes even within hours. Thus a child may go from the qi level one day to the nutritive-qi level the next. In such cases the tongue will change from being slightly red with a thick yellow coating (qi level) to being red or dark red without coating (nutritive-qi level). The former is shown in PLATE 41, and the latter in PLATE 42.

Finally, children are frequently given antibiotics during acute febrile diseases, the side-effects of which clearly show on the tongue. In children antibiotics usually cause the coating to fall off or become thinner in patches, so that the tongue becomes partially peeled. This indicates injury to the Stomach yin. When the tongue shows such signs following or during the administration of antibiotics, any herbal formula used should be modified to include herbs that nourish Stomach yin such as Radix Pseudostellariae Heterophyllae *(tai zi shen),* Radix Dioscoreae Oppositae *(shan yao)* or Rhizoma Polygonati Odorati *(yu zhu).*

Apart from the changes in the tongue brought about by invasions of external wind, certain children's tongues show hereditary traits. A fairly common one is the so-called geographic tongue. This is a tongue that is peeled in patches, with the peeled patches having quite defined white borders (PLATES 10 & 44). This indicates constitutional Stomach yin deficiency and is frequently seen in such children's allergic diseases as allergic asthma and atopic eczema. A study of 17 children with peeled tongues showed that 10 had geographic tongues: of these 10, five had an allergic constitution and were suffering from allergic asthma and atopic eczema.[4]

Children's tongues also show signs of heat with red points more often than do adults (PLATE 41). This is typical as red points reflect the arousal of pathological ministerial fire, which is naturally very strong in children. The clinical significance of red points depends on their distribution and is the same as for adults, i.e., Liver fire if they are on the sides, Stomach fire if they are on the edges in the central section, Heart fire if they are on the tip, and Bladder or Intestinal damp-heat if they are on the root. However, many children often have red points all over the tongue. In acute cases this is usually due to Lung heat, while in chronic cases it is generally due to heat in the Stomach and Intestines.

NOTES

1. Fan De-Rong, "Analysis of Tongue Picture and Pathology of Patients with Stomach Carcinoma." *Journal of Traditional Chinese Medicine (Zhong yi za zhi)* 32, no. 10 (1991): 34.

2. Qian Zong-Que, "Tongue Examination in 122 Cases of Bone Fractures." *Journal of Traditional Chinese Medicine (Zhong yi za zhi)* 27, no. 11 (1986): 41.

3. Sun Yuan Qin, "Observation of Tongue Appearance in 2721 Healthy Children." *Journal of Traditional Chinese Medicine (Zhong yi za zhi)* 27, no.3 (1986): 57.

4. Gansu College of Traditional Chinese Medicine, "Patterns and Treatment of Geographic Tongue in Children." *Journal of Traditional Chinese Medicine (Zhong yi za zhi)* 33, no. 4 (1992): 40.

9
Case Histories

PLATE 1: Woman, Age 34

TONGUE SIGNS

Body color: normal
Body shape: normal, except for slight swelling of the sides
Coating: thick, dark yellow

CASE HISTORY

This patient was in relatively good health and suffered primarily from frontal headaches, stiff neck and poor digestion. The pulse was weak, especially in the right, middle position.

DIAGNOSIS

The dark yellow, thick coating indicates retention of food in the Stomach giving, rise to some heat. The problem is confined to the Stomach as the remainder of the tongue is normal, except for the slight swelling of the sides, which denotes slight Spleen qi deficiency. This tongue is shown here as an example of coating with root, in contrast to PLATE 20, which shows a coating without root.

Whenever the tongue body is nearly normal and the coating has root — no matter how dark or thick the coating — the condition is not serious, the prognosis is good, and the condition should be easy to cure (which was true in this case).

PLATE 2: Man, Age 65

TONGUE SIGNS

Body color: red, redder on the sides
Body shape: long, slightly swollen, more on the right side

Coating: thin, yellow and wet coating in the Lung area (behind the tip)

CASE HISTORY

This patient suffered from osteoarthritis of both hips and hypertension for two years. The pulse was full, wiry, rapid and deep.

DIAGNOSIS

The red tongue body, which is redder on the sides, denotes the presence of heat in the Liver, i.e., Liver fire. The long body also indicates heat, and the slight swelling on the right side also denotes Liver fire. This is confirmed by the rapid and wiry pulse, which suggests interior heat associated with the Liver fire. The hypertension is caused, in this case, by the rising of Liver fire. The slight swelling of the whole tongue is caused by the accumulation of dampness from Spleen qi deficiency. The thin, yellow coating in the Lung area reflects the long-term retention of dampness and phlegm in the Lungs; this is usually due to a past cold or influenza which was not properly treated (or treated with antibiotics), leading to the accumulation of dampness and phlegm in the Lungs. Such patients may not be aware of any problem in the chest, but are prone to further attacks of external pathogenic factors.

PLATE 3: Woman, Age 76

TONGUE SIGNS

Body color: deep red, many raised red spots
Body shape: short (contracted)
Coating: completely peeled (no coating), dry

CASE HISTORY

This patient had been suffering from Parkinson's disease for over ten years. She was very thin and her skin was dry. The pulse was extremely thin, floating and empty.

DIAGNOSIS

This is a very extreme case of yin deficiency of the Kidneys. The deep red tongue body, the total absence of coating, the raised red spots and the dryness all reflect a severe exhaustion of Kidney yin with blazing deficiency heat. The yin deficiency is also confirmed by her thinness and dry skin. A tongue such as this always points to a poor prognosis, and the condition must be regarded as incurable.

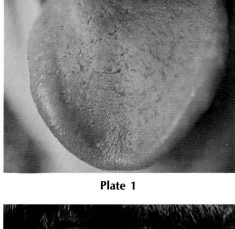

Plate 1

Plate 1 — Normal body except for slight swelling of the sides; a thick, dark yellow coating.

Plate 2 — Long, slightly swollen and red (especially on the sides); more swollen on the right side; a thin, yellow and wet coating in the Lung area (behind the tip).

Plate 3 — Short, dry, deep red; many raised red spots; completely peeled.

Plate 4 — Red with points on the left side; a thick, yellow, greasy and sticky coating.

Plate 5 — Red and swollen; a rootless, moldy and partially peeled coating.

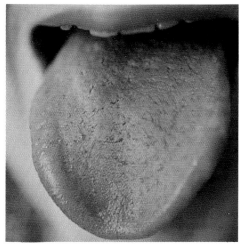

Plate 2

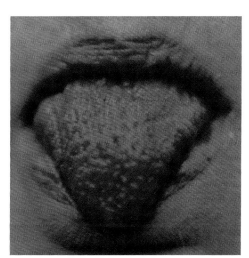

Plate 3

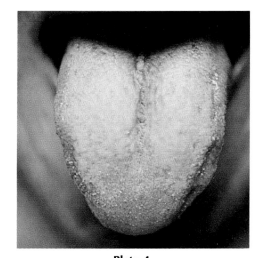

Plate 4

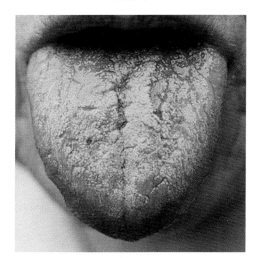

Plate 5

Plate 6 — Pale and swollen with some cracks; a thin, white and dry coating.

Plate 7 — Thin, dark red, slightly flaccid; redder and slightly swollen on the sides; a crack in the center to the tip; slight swelling of the chest area; a thin, white coating.

Plate 8 — Swollen sides and a crack in the center to the tip; swelling on both sides of the crack and prickles inside it; a sticky and dirty coating.

Plate 9 — Pale, swollen tongue with a wet coating.

Plate 10 — Normal except for red points and a thin, white coating on the right side.

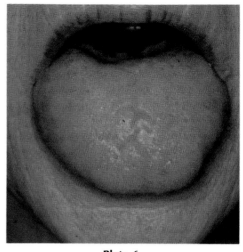

Plate 6

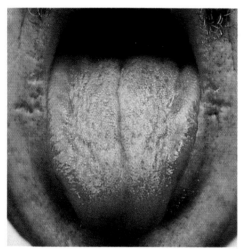

Plate 7

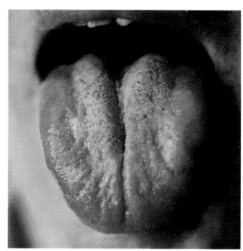

Plate 8

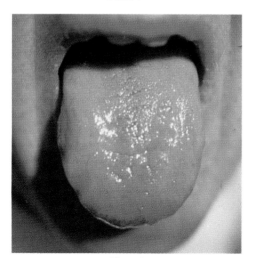

Plate 9

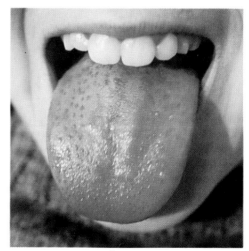

Plate 10

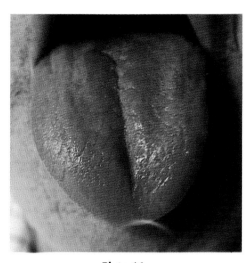

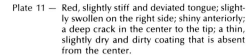

Plate 11 — Red, slightly stiff and deviated tongue; slightly swollen on the right side; shiny anteriorly; a deep crack in the center to the tip; a thin, slightly dry and dirty coating that is absent from the center.

Plate 12 — Red, swollen (especially just behind the tip and on the sides); red spots on the root; slight cracks on the sides; a dip in the Lung area; increased moisture on the sides and especially in the dip; no coating in the center and a yellow coating on the root.

Plate 13 — Dark red with red spots between the tip and center; orange sides (especially the right side); many "ice floe" cracks; no coating.

Plate 14 — Bluish-purple with pale and concave red spots; teeth marks; dry, dirty coating.

Plate 15 — Pale (except for a red tip) and swollen; pale red concave spots around the center; raised red points anteriorly; a coating that is yellow in the center and white elsewhere.

Plate 11

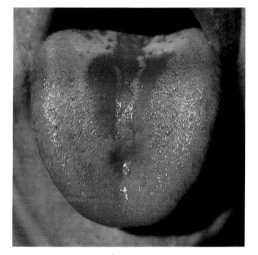

Plate 12

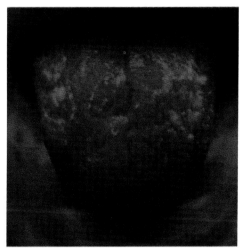

Plate 13

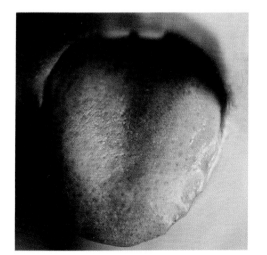

Plate 14

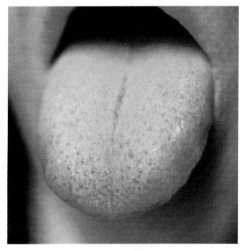

Plate 15

Plate 16 — Pale and slightly swollen; pale red points on the left side; wet sides; a thin, yellow and dirty coating.

Plate 17 — Slightly swollen sides; a thin and yellow coating that is without root and is peeled in patches.

Plate 18 — Red with a redder tip; swollen; curled over; a sticky, yellow and dry coating.

Plate 19 — Deep red to reddish-purple; redder and swollen anteriorly; points on the sides; peeled, except for a thin white coating on the sides.

Plate 20 — Slightly red in the center; rootless and peeled coating in the center; swollen; thin, yellow coating between the tip and the center.

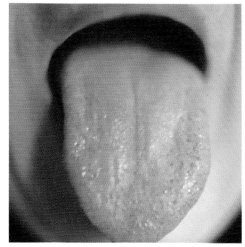

Plate 16

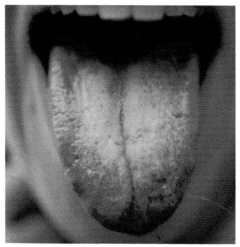

Plate 17

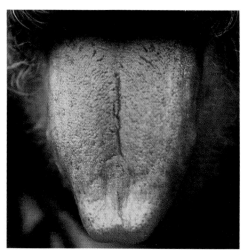

Plate 18

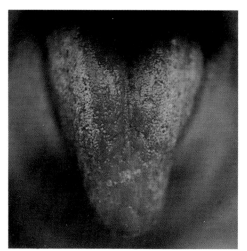

Plate 19

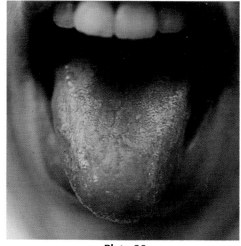

Plate 20

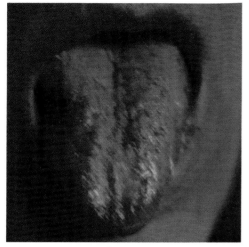

Plate 21

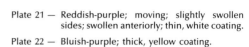

Plate 21 — Reddish-purple; moving; slightly swollen sides; swollen anteriorly; thin, white coating.

Plate 22 — Bluish-purple; thick, yellow coating.

Plate 23 — Deep red; sides redder; swollen anteriorly and on the sides; white, powder-like, dry and rootless coating.

Plate 24 — Deep red; deep central crack to the tip with many other cracks radiating out from it; swollen alongside the central crack; peeled.

Plate 25 — Normal color; wide crack in the center that does not extend to the tip; slight cracks on the sides; no coating.

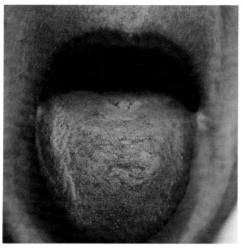

Plate 22

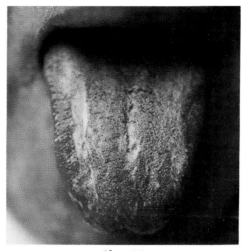

Plate 23

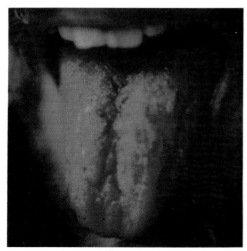

Plate 24

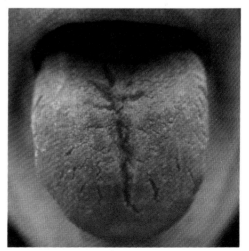

Plate 25

Plate 26 — Red (especially the tip); crack in the center reaching to the tip; other small cracks; peeled; the tip is especially dry while the root is wet.

Plate 27 — Reddish-purple; slightly swollen; crack in the center extending to the tip; slightly stiff; yellow prickles inside the crack; dry, thin and rootless coating that is yellow on the root.

Plate 28 — Red; thick, yellow, black and dry coating; scattered white, moldy coating on the left side.

Plate 29 — Normal color; central crack; cracks on the sides; scattered cracks elsewhere; no coating.

Plate 30 — Bluish-purple; slightly swollen; crack in the center; thin, white coating.

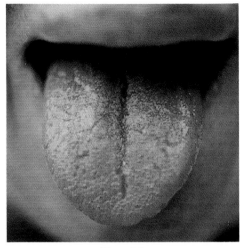

Plate 26

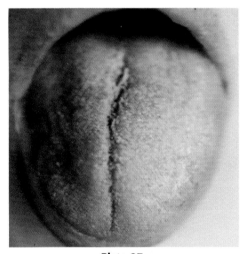

Plate 27

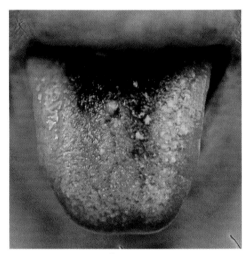

Plate 28

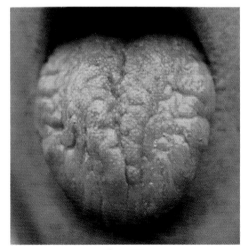

Plate 29

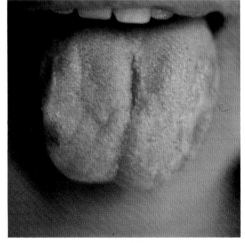

Plate 30

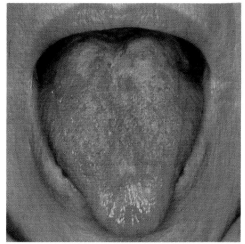

Plate 31

Plate 31 — Reddish-purple; red tip; swollen (especially on the tip); stiff; thin, white, rootless coating; peeled patches on the root.

Plate 32 — Normal except for a swelling superficially on the right half.

Plate 33 — Slightly red left side and tip; slightly swollen left side; yellow and slippery coating on the left side.

Plate 34 — Very swollen (especially on the sides); many deep cracks on the sides; dry, powder-like and rootless coating.

Plate 35 — Same patient two years later (note absence of cracks).

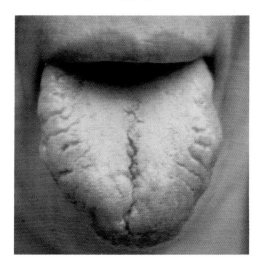

Plate 32

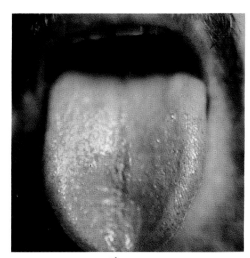

Plate 33

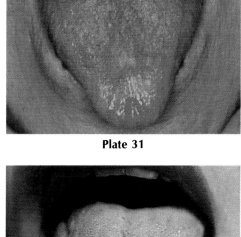

Plate 34

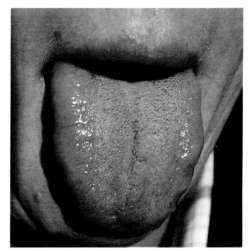

Plate 35

Plate 36 — [1 of 3] Normal color; red points on the tip and sides; yellow, sticky coating.

Plate 37 — [2 of 3] Same as Plate 36 with a more slippery coating.

Plate 38 — [3 of 3] Normal color; pale red points (not so raised); thin, white coating.

Plate 39 — Red with slightly purple sides; purple and distended vein on the right side.

Plate 40 — Normal underside of the tongue.

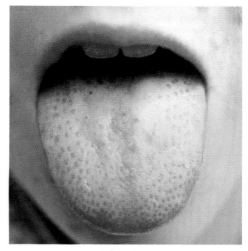

Plate 36

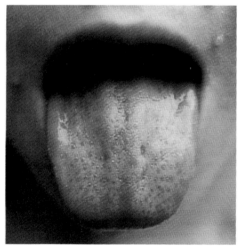

Plate 37

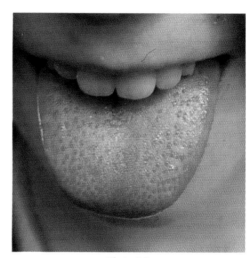

Plate 38

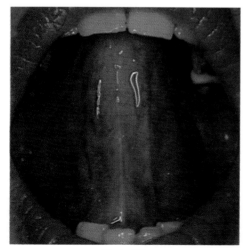

Plate 39

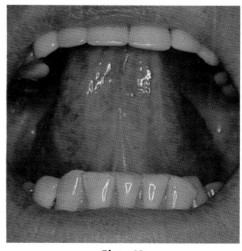

Plate 40

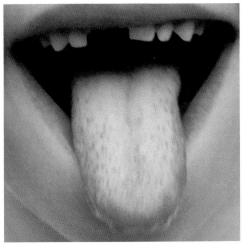

Plate 41

Plate 41 — Red, especially in the front part which is swollen; red points around the center; thick, yellow, with root.

Plate 42 — Same patient two years later (note absence of coating in the front).

Plate 43 — Pale, but red on the root; swollen; thin, white coating except on root, which is peeled.

Plate 44 — Normal color with red points on front part; tooth-marked; peeled in patches ("geographic").

Plate 45 — Pale; swollen, tooth-marked; crack in middle; coating is sticky and white overall, but slightly yellow in the center toward the root.

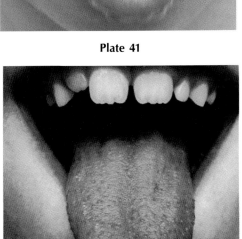

Plate 42

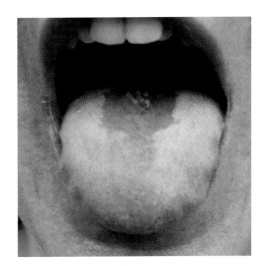

Plate 43

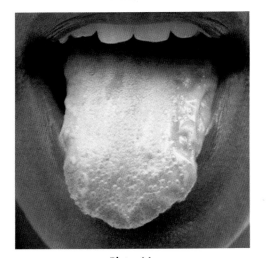

Plate 44

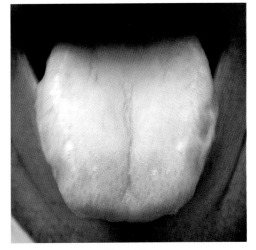

Plate 45

Plate 46 — Pale; swollen, more so in the front; tooth-marked; sticky white coating.

Plate 47 — Red; tip red with red points; stiff; thick, yellow, very dry coating.

Plate 48 — Red; slightly swollen sides; scattered cracks; peeled.

Plate 49 — Reddish purple; red points in front; central crack; tooth-marked; sticky white coating (yellow inside crack); peeled in patches, especially toward front.

Plate 50 — Slightly pale, especially sides; slightly swollen, more so in front; slightly sticky coating.

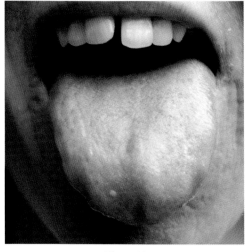

Plate 46

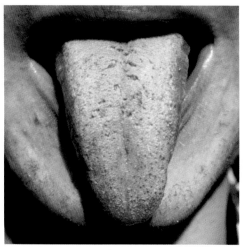

Plate 47

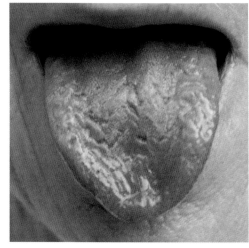

Plate 48

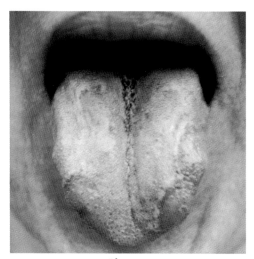

Plate 49

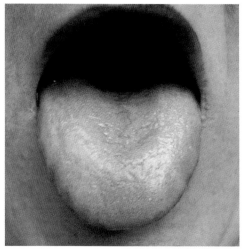

Plate 50

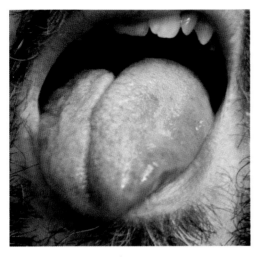

Plate 51

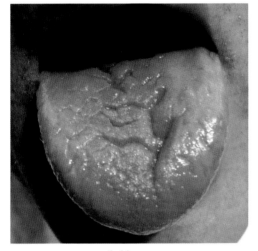

Plate 52

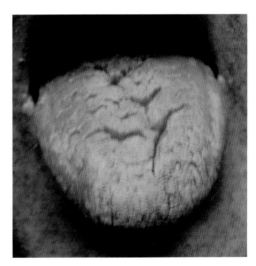

Plate 53

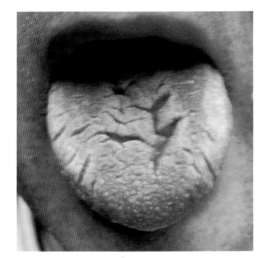

Plate 54

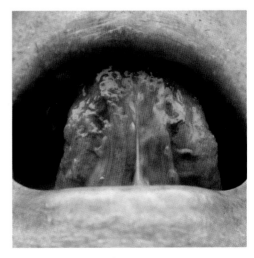

Plate 55

Plate 56 — Pale; wet; slightly swollen; no coating.

Plate 57 — Normal with red root; slightly dry; slightly swollen, especially in front; transverse cracks on the edges; peeled in patches ("geographic").

Plate 58 — Same patient three months later: root is less red, body is less dry, cracks are less deep; some coating has returned on root.

Plate 59 — Reddish purple; dry; long, deep cracks; only patches of thick, yellow, rootless coating.

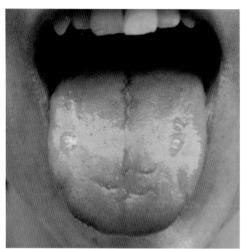

Plate 56

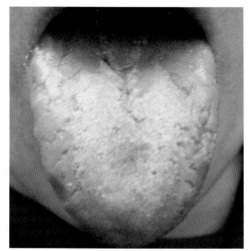

Plate 57

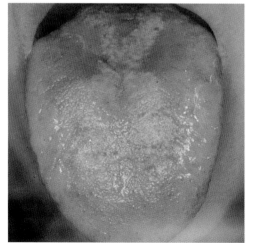

Plate 58

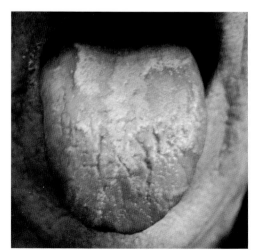

Plate 59

PLATE 4: Man, Age 25

TONGUE SIGNS

Body color: red, with points on the left side
Body shape: normal
Coating: thick, yellow, greasy and sticky

CASE HISTORY

This patient suffered from hypochondriac pain, constipation, dizziness, thirst, a bitter taste in the mouth, and irritability. The pulse was full and wiry.

DIAGNOSIS

All the symptoms point to Liver fire. This is confirmed by the tongue, since the tongue body is red and there are red points on the left side, which is associated with the Liver. Since there is a coating, it is excess heat. Furthermore, because the coating is thick, greasy and sticky, it indicates that there is also dampness or phlegm affecting the Gallbladder. We can deduce that the Gallbladder is also affected from the presence of a thick coating, which signifies a problem in a yang Organ. This is a coating with root.

PLATE 5: Woman, Age 80

TONGUE SIGNS

Body color: red
Body shape: swollen
Coating: rootless, moldy, partially peeled

CASE HISTORY

This patient suffered from rheumatism of the wrists and knees. Apart from this, she was relatively healthy.

DIAGNOSIS

This tongue clearly shows heat and deficiency of Stomach yin. The swelling of the body is, in this case, due to heat. The partially peeled coating indicates Stomach yin deficiency. The "moldy" coating (only slightly moldy in this patient) suggests that there is heat in the Stomach (in this case from Stomach yin deficiency), which evaporates the Stomach fluids and causes them to go up to the tongue. The moldy coating looks like crumbled beancurd, curdled milk or porridge.

Even though the tongue shows an advanced pathology of the Stomach, this patient is relatively healthy. This apparent contradiction can be explained by the age of the patient. At an advanced age the yin usually becomes deficient (in this case, more the Stomach yin) and the tongue will show certain changes, while the patient is often free of symptoms.

PLATE 6: Woman, Age 65

TONGUE SIGNS

Body color: pale
Body shape: swollen, with some cracks
Coating: thin, white and dry

CASE HISTORY

This patient suffered from chronic asthma, with particular difficulty in inhalation, for over thirty years. She had considerable mucus in the chest, which was occasionally coughed up. The mucus was white and watery. The pulse was weak, especially in the proximal position.

DIAGNOSIS

The pale and swollen tongue body denotes a deficiency of Spleen yang with accumulation of dampness. Kidney yang is also deficient, as shown by the weakness of the pulse at the proximal position. The deficiency of Kidney yang can also be deduced from the long duration of the condition and the nature of the problem. Any long-standing deficiency of the Spleen can, over time, lead to a deficiency of the Kidneys. In the case of very chronic asthma in an elderly person in particular, the Kidneys are almost certain to be affected. This is also confirmed by the fact that inhalation is more difficult than exhalation: this is due to the impairment of the Kidneys' function of grasping the qi.

The patient's tongue coating is dry and has some cracks, which reflects the long-standing deficiency of yang. When yang qi is very deficient over a long period of time, it cannot move the fluids, which then do not reach the tongue; hence the dry and slightly cracked tongue body. A pale and dry tongue can also indicate blood deficiency. How do we know in this case that it is due to yang deficiency? Because the tongue body is quite swollen, which denotes accumulation of dampness caused by yang deficiency of the Spleen. In the case of blood deficiency the tongue body would either be thin or of normal size.

PLATE 7: Man, Age 67

TONGUE SIGNS

Body color: dark red, redder on the sides
Body shape: thin, sides slightly swollen, crack in the center to the tip, slightly swollen in the chest area (between the tip and center all across the tongue), slightly flaccid
Coating: thin and white

CASE HISTORY

This patient suffered from chronic lower back pain and tinnitus. The pulse was full, rapid and wiry.

DIAGNOSIS

The dark red tongue body indicates the presence of heat. The sides are redder and slightly swollen: this shows that the heat is in the Liver. This is confirmed by the rapid and wiry pulse. There is a crack in the center to the tip, which indicates that Liver fire has been transmitted to the Heart, giving rise to Heart fire. The body is thin because the heat has begun to injure and dry up the body fluids, but this has not yet resulted in yin deficiency. The slight swelling between the tip and the center denotes stagnation of qi in the chest (presumably from emotional problems, as there is also Heart fire). The swelling in this area causes the crack to deviate, which shows that the stagnation of qi in the chest has constricted the Heart.

PLATE 8: Man, Age 62

TONGUE SIGNS

Body color: normal
Body shape: swollen on the sides, crack in the center to the tip with swelling on both sides
Coating: sticky and dirty with prickles inside the central crack

CASE HISTORY

This patient suffered from epigastric pain, indigestion and rheumatic pain in the wrists and knees. The pulse was deep and weak, except for the Heart pulse, which was overflowing but empty.

DIAGNOSIS

In this case the body shape and coating are primary in relation to the body color, which does not show pathological changes. The swelling of the sides indicates a long-standing deficiency of Spleen qi, which is unable to transform and transport the fluids. The central crack down to the tip shows a constitutional weakness of the Heart, and the swelling around it suggests that the Heart qi has been further disrupted by emotional trauma. The swelling on either side of the central crack reflects that the heart is enlarged. This is also borne out by the overflowing and empty Heart pulse, which indicates that the Heart qi is weak (hence the empty pulse) and that the patient is driving himself too hard and has some emotional problems (hence the overflowing pulse).

The dirty coating and prickles inside the central crack show that there has been retention of food in the Stomach for a long time, which has now been transformed into Stomach phlegm and fire. The phlegm is reflected in the stickiness of the coating.

In sum, both the Stomach and Spleen have been deficient for a long time, which has led to the accumulation of dampness and the formation of phlegm and fire in the Stomach. Eventually, the phlegm and fire could produce mental symptoms, "misting" the spirit. This is shown by the presence of prickles inside the central crack, which is related to the Heart.

PLATE 9: Woman, Age 51

TONGUE SIGNS

Body color: pale
Body shape: swollen
Coating: wet

CASE HISTORY

This patient suffered from persistent shaking of the head, which started two years previously. She also had slight palpitations, insomnia and frequent urination, also at night. The pulse was weak and deep. The biomedical diagnosis for her condition was Parkinson's disease.

DIAGNOSIS

The pale tongue body indicates deficiency of yang, which is confirmed by the swelling of the body and the wetness of the coating. In this case the deficient yang qi has led to the accumulation of dampness, as shown by the swollen and wet tongue body. The deficiency of yang is of the Spleen and Kidneys, judging by the pulse and the frequent urination. The deficiency of Spleen yang has also led to the Spleen being unable to generate enough blood, and therefore to blood deficiency. This is manifested in the palpitations and insomnia. The deficiency of blood, in turn, has led to a rising of Liver wind, which is the cause of the shaking. It is important to note that this is deficiency wind because it arises from deficiency of blood. In this case, judging by the pulse and tongue, the condition is primarily one of deficiency and therefore calls for tonification of the Spleen and Kidneys.

PLATE 10: Girl, Age 10

TONGUE SIGNS

Body color: normal, with red points on the right side
Body shape: normal
Coating: thin white coating on the right side

CASE HISTORY

This child was suffering at the time from an acute upper respiratory tract infection with sore throat and pain in one ear.

DIAGNOSIS

This tongue is a clear example of external attack of wind-heat at the lesser yang stage. In the lesser yang pattern there is typically a thin white coating on the right side only, as in this case. In addition, there are red points on the right side, which indicates that the heat is beginning to proceed into the interior.

PLATE 11: Man, Age 64

TONGUE SIGNS

Body color: red, shiny anteriorly
Body shape: slightly stiff and deviated, deep crack in the center to the tip, right side slightly swollen
Coating: thin, slightly dry and dirty, no coating in the center

CASE HISTORY

This patient suffered from chronic rheumatoid arthritis, mostly affecting the shoulders, elbows and wrists. Four years previously he had a stomach ulcer which perforated. The pulse was mostly wiry and rapid, less so on the right hand side, which was slightly weak and floating in the middle position.

DIAGNOSIS

The red tongue body indicates the presence of heat, in this case at the blood level, as the tongue is also slightly dry. The slight stiffness and deviation of the tongue denote the presence (or the beginning) of Liver wind, probably stirred by heat in the blood. The absence of coating in the center indicates deficiency of Stomach yin, and the deep central crack to the tip denotes a constitutional weakness of the Heart, further aggravated during his life by the presence of heat. The slight swelling of the right side indicates that there is more heat on that side. This is an example of an excess type of swelling because the tongue body is red. Although the pain in the shoulders, elbows and wrists would be considered a painful obstruction *(bi)* disorder due to invasion of the channels by external damp-cold, in this case it is also influenced by the internal condition. The presence of heat in the blood and slight Liver wind suggests that the blood is "stirred" in the blood vessels; this predisposes the vessels and channels to attack by external pathogenic factors. Because of the heat in the blood, the external pathogenic factors will readily transform into heat, which is what happened in this patient. The stomach problem (ulcer) is clearly reflected in both the tongue and pulse and manifests as Stomach yin deficiency.

PLATE 12: Man, Age 66

TONGUE SIGNS

Body color: red, with red spots on the root
Body shape: swollen, especially just behind the tip and on the sides, slight cracks on the sides, dip in the Lung area

Coating: no coating in the center, slightly wet on the sides, yellow coating on the root, very wet within the dip in the Lung area

CASE HISTORY

This patient had been suffering from emphysema and asthma for the past ten years, with shortness of breath and pain in the chest. Many years previously he had pleurisy and a duodenal ulcer. The pulse was rapid and slippery, but rather weak on the right side.

DIAGNOSIS

This tongue reflects a complicated pathology. It clearly shows a combination of excess and deficiency conditions. The red body indicates heat, which is confirmed by the rapid pulse. The swelling, particularly in the Lung area, denotes the retention of dampness and phlegm in the Lungs. This is confirmed by the slippery pulse, and also very clearly shown by the large dip in the Lung area, with accumulation of fluid inside. The swelling and slight cracks on the sides denote the long-standing condition of Spleen qi deficiency, the Spleen being unable to transform fluids, which accumulate in the form of dampness and phlegm in the Lungs. There is a saying in Chinese medicine, "The Spleen produces phlegm, the Lungs store it." The peeled coating in the center extending to the root clearly indicates yin deficiency of the Stomach affecting the Intestines, which is confirmed by the red spots on the root. These signs also reflect the presence of heat and stagnation in the Intestines, which was the cause of the duodenal ulcer in the past. The heat in the lower burner (Intestines) is also confirmed by the yellow coating and red spots on the root.

In summary, this tongue shows a combination of excess and deficiency. The deficiency conditions include Spleen qi deficiency and Stomach yin deficiency. The excess conditions include the retention of dampness and phlegm in the Lungs, and heat and stagnation in the Intestines.

PLATE 13: Woman, Age 41

TONGUE SIGNS

Body color: dark red, red spots between the tip and center, sides slightly orange-colored, particularly on the right
Body shape: many cracks of the "ice floe" type
Coating: no coating

CASE HISTORY

This patient suffered from migraine headaches at the temples, extreme fatigue, anxiety and indigestion. Her hair had been falling out for the past two years, and she suffered from constipation. The pulse was thin and slightly rapid.

DIAGNOSIS

The dark red tongue body without coating and the many cracks clearly denote deficiency of yin, in this case of both the Stomach and Kidneys. The slight orange color on the sides suggests a severe, long-standing deficiency of blood, which has become deficiency of yin. The red spots between the tip and the center indicate blood stasis in the chest. The deficiency of Kidney yin caused the rising of Liver yang, as evidenced by the migraine headaches at the temples. The extreme fatigue, loss of hair and anxiety all reflect deficiency of Kidney yin. This is a rather severe condition (red body without coating, with cracks), especially since the patient is young.

PLATE 14: Woman, Age 52

TONGUE SIGNS

Body color: bluish purple with pale and concave red spots
Body shape: tooth-marked
Coating: dry, dirty

CASE HISTORY

This patient suffered from chronic frontal headaches, tension and stiffness of the neck muscles and hypertension. The pulse was thin, slow and weak.

DIAGNOSIS

The bluish purple color of the tongue body indicates stagnation of cold in the interior from severe and long-standing deficiency of yang. This tongue must have been pale to begin with and, as the deficiency of yang worsened, there was some stasis, which caused the tongue to become bluish purple. The dryness in this case derives from deficiency of yang qi, which is unable to move the fluids. The concave, pale red spots indicate cold in the interior. The tooth marks denote deficiency of Spleen qi, while the dirty coating reflects the retention of food resulting from Spleen qi deficiency. In sum, this patient suffers from a severe and long-standing deficiency of the Stomach and Spleen, leading to blood stasis and interior cold. The frontal headaches are due to deficiency of the Stomach.

It is interesting in this case that the patient's hypertension is caused by the blood stasis from Internal cold, and not by the rising of Liver yang, as in most cases.

PLATE 15: Woman, Age 28

TONGUE SIGNS

Body color: pale, except red on the tip, pale red concave spots around the center, raised red points anteriorly
Body shape: swollen
Coating: yellow in the center, white elsewhere

CASE HISTORY

This patient suffered from fatigue, loose stools, depression and a feeling of heaviness in the head. In the past she suffered sunstroke in India, which caused high fever and delirium. The pulse was weak.

DIAGNOSIS

The pale and swollen tongue body points to a deficiency of Spleen yang with retention of dampness. The pale red spots around the center denote the presence of cold in the Stomach. This is in contradiction to the thin yellow coating, which signifies heat. This could simply be due to a temporary condition of slight heat, which in turn could be caused by dietary factors or smoking. The raised red points in the front part correspond to the upper burner area and are related to the sunstroke which she had previously suffered. Heat invaded the upper burner, and in particular the Pericardium, causing delirium. This is still reflected on the tongue tip.

PLATE 16: Woman, Age 52

TONGUE SIGNS

Body color: pale, with pale red points on the left side
Body shape: slightly swollen on the left side
Coating: thin, yellow and dirty, wet on the sides

CASE HISTORY

This patient suffered from chronic neck pain and lower back pain for over fifteen years. Biomedical investigations revealed severe osteoarthritis of the cervical vertebrae. She also suffered from severe dizziness and fatigue. In the past she had several falls and accidents. She had undergone a hysterectomy (for heavy periods) fifteen years previously. Ten years previously she had an acute episode of very high temperature and severe headache which went undiagnosed, but which resembled meningitis. This was followed by a feeling of weakness and near-paralysis of the left side, symptoms which recovered spontaneously after a few weeks. The pulse was weak, particularly so in both proximal positions.

DIAGNOSIS

The pale tongue with wet sides indicates a deficiency of Spleen yang, which is unable to transport and transform the fluids. There is also deficiency of Kidney yang manifested by the severe dizziness and the weak pulse in both Kidney positions. The Kidneys control the bones; in this case the Kidney deficiency is a contributing factor to the cervical arthritis. The neck pain is a form of painful obstruction *(bi)* disorder from damp-cold. The accidents and falls are also contributory factors, as they cause stagnation of qi in the muscles, which would aggravate the pain. Finally, it has been my experience that a hysterectomy often causes severe stiffness and pain in the back of the neck.

The tongue contains contradictory features because the body is pale (denoting cold) while the coating is yellow (denoting heat). There can be several explanations for such contradictory signs, but in this case it simply means that although the general condition is one of cold and deficiency of yang, there is also slight heat in the Stomach, as indicated by the yellow coating. This can occur when a chronic deficiency of Spleen qi or Spleen yang leads to long-standing retention of food, which in turn can create slight heat in the Stomach. This is apparently what happened here.

The swelling and pale red points on the left side signify a weakness and malnourishment of the channels on that side. This stems from the episode of high temperature, which burned the body fluids on the left side and led to the temporary paralysis. Even though she recovered from this, a slight weakness of the left arm and leg remains, showing on the tongue as swelling and pale red points on the left side. Upon needling, the "arrival of qi" is also slower on the left side. The deficiency of the Spleen (which controls the muscles) would contribute to this state of weakness in the muscles of her left side.

PLATE 17: Woman, Age 38

TONGUE SIGNS

Body color: normal
Body shape: normal, except for very slightly swollen sides and a crack down the center
Coating: thin and yellow, without root, peeled in patches

CASE HISTORY

This patient suffered from hypochondriac pain, abdominal distension, some epigastric pain, slight thirst and dry stools. The pulse was thin and slightly weak and floating in the right middle position.

DIAGNOSIS

This tongue indicates a clear deficiency of Stomach yin because of its rootless coating, which is peeled in places. Most of the symptoms reflect the deficiency of Stomach yin (thirst, dry stools, epigastric pain, slightly weak and floating Stomach pulse).

PLATE 18: Man, Age 23

TONGUE SIGNS

Body color: red, tip redder
Body shape: tip rolled over and swollen
Coating: sticky, yellow and dry

CASE HISTORY

This patient had been suffering from recurring boils in the elbow region, which were very hot, red and painful. There was no other complaint and the pulse was rapid and full.

DIAGNOSIS

This is a good example of how the tongue can reveal a great deal of information about the condition and cause of a disease even in a patient with very few presenting symptoms. In this case all the signs on the tongue point to heat: the red body and the dry, yellow coating. The reddish tip, which is swollen and rolls over, clearly shows the presence of Heart fire. This is probably caused by emotional problems, as is often the case. The yellow, sticky and dry coating denotes phlegm and fire in the Stomach and Intestines. This is obviously the cause of the recurrent painful boils, which occur along the Large Intestine channel in this patient.

PLATE 19: Woman, Age 61

TONGUE SIGNS

Body color: deep red tending to reddish purple, tip redder, with points on the sides
Body shape: swollen anteriorly (including the tip)
Coating: peeled, except for a thin white coating on the sides.

CASE HISTORY

This patient suffered from severe bronchial asthma for thirty years. She had a cough productive of a thick yellow sputum. Inhalation was more difficult than exhalation, and breathing was more difficult when lying down. She did not sleep well and her appetite was poor. She also suffered from lower back pain and often felt hot in the evenings. At the time this photograph was taken she was suffering from acute bronchitis. The pulse was slippery and rapid.

DIAGNOSIS

This patient was treated over a long course of time, at some points in which there was no thin white coating on the sides. This clearly reflects an acute attack of wind-cold or wind-heat. The deep red color of the tongue body and the complete absence of coating (at other times) indicate severe deficiency of Kidney yin with deficiency heat. The swelling of the front part of the tongue and the bright red color of the tip indicate the retention of phlegm in the Lungs as well as the presence of deficiency heat in the Heart. The presence of phlegm is also indicated by the slippery pulse. The phlegm is formed as a result of the dysfunction in the Spleen's transformation of fluids, hence the lack of appetite (from Spleen qi deficiency).

All the other symptoms are caused by the deficiency of Kidney yin (lower back pain, difficulty of inhalation, feeling hot in the evenings) and the presence of deficiency heat in the Heart (insomnia). The red points on the sides and the slight reddish purple color of the tongue body also indicate blood stasis in the Liver.

PLATE 20: Woman, Age 37

TONGUE SIGNS

Body color: normal, slightly red in the center
Body shape: swollen
Coating: rootless and peeled in the center; thin, yellow coating between tip and center

CASE HISTORY

This patient suffered from severe migraine headaches with pain at the temple since the birth of her first child. She often vomited during the migraine attacks. She also suffered from occasional severe abdominal pain followed by diarrhea. The pulse was weak and floating and both proximal positions were deep and weak, while the left middle position was wiry.

DIAGNOSIS

This tongue primarily shows a severe deficiency of Stomach yin because the coating is patchy and looks scattered on the tongue surface, rather than growing out of it. Furthermore, there is no coating at all in the center and toward the root. All these signs clearly indicate severe deficiency of Stomach yin. This condition also affects the Intestines because the peeling of the coating extends toward the root. We can also deduce that there is Kidney yin deficiency, partly because we know that Stomach yin deficiency often precedes Kidney yin deficiency (and this tongue reflects an advanced stage of Stomach yin deficiency), and partly because the pulse is deep and weak at both Kidney positions. We can further deduce the presence of Kidney deficiency from the history: her migraines started after the birth of her first child, which often happens when Kidney qi is weak and is further weakened by pregnancy and childbirth.

The Kidney yin deficiency here has clearly induced the rising of Liver yang, as the migraine headaches at the temple show. The stagnant Liver qi has also invaded the Stomach, causing vomiting, and the Spleen, causing the abdominal pain and diarrhea. Furthermore, there is also some dampness (derived from Spleen qi deficiency) indicated by the swollen tongue body. The thin, yellow coating between the tip and center of the tongue denotes retention of phlegm in the Lungs as a result of a past cold or influenza, which was either not treated properly, or treated with antibiotics.

PLATE 21: Man, Age 67

TONGUE SIGNS

Body color: reddish purple
Body shape: tip swollen, moving, slightly swollen sides, swollen anteriorly
Coating: thin, white

CASE HISTORY

This is a good example of the prognostic value of tongue diagnosis. The patient had very few symptoms other than occasional pain in the chest. He sought acupuncture treatment only once or twice a year whenever he had a cold, flu or sore throat. His tongue and pulse, however, clearly indicated a dangerous condition. His pulse was full, wiry, rapid and hasty (stopping at irregular intervals). He subsequently died of myocardial infarction.

DIAGNOSIS

The reddish purple color definitely indicates blood stasis with heat. The swelling of the sides and tip, together with the redder color of the tip, show that there is heat and stagnation in the Liver and Heart. This is also indicated by the rapid, wiry and hasty pulse. The moving tongue body (which accounts for the photograph being slightly out of focus) signifies that Liver fire has given rise to Liver wind. The swelling anteriorly also suggests that there is severe blood stasis in the chest. All of these factors (heat, blood stasis and internal wind) caused the myocardial infarction.

PLATE 22: Woman, Age 56

TONGUE SIGNS

Body color: bluish purple
Body shape: unremarkable
Coating: thick, yellow

CASE HISTORY

This patient had been suffering from multiple sclerosis for twenty-five years. She was still walking, but very slowly and dragging one foot. One foot was dropped and both were swollen. Her hand movement was difficult and she was incapable of fine movements, such as those needed for sewing. She had cramps and pain in the legs, which were purple and very cold. She also suffered from numbness of the limbs, dizziness, a feeling of "muzziness" in her head and blurred vision. The pulse was slow and choppy.

DIAGNOSIS

The bluish purple color is due to stagnation of cold in the interior. This patient had obviously suffered from yang deficiency for a long time, and the resulting interior cold had led to stagnation of blood. The long-standing deficiency of yang had affected the Kidneys and Liver, thus weakening the bones and sinews, a cause of her multiple sclerosis. An additional factor was that of phlegm, as evidenced by the thick coating. Phlegm is often a factor in multiple sclerosis and accounts for the symptoms of numbness, dizziness and blurred vision.

The yellow coating is an apparent contradiction because it indicates heat, while every other sign points to cold: the bluish purple tongue, the slow pulse and her feeling of cold. The deficiency of Spleen qi (which caused the phlegm) led to poor digestion and retention of food. Because this condition was of long duration, the retention of food in the Stomach gave rise to heat.

PLATE 23: Man, Age 59

TONGUE SIGNS

Body color: deep red, sides redder
Body shape: swollen anteriorly and on the sides
Coating: white, powder-like, dry and rootless

CASE HISTORY

This patient suffered from chronic asthma since the age of three. The shortness of breath was worse on exhalation. He also suffered from hypochondriac pain and dream-disturbed sleep. Two years previously he had suffered from fluid in the abdomen. Upon questioning, he also revealed that he suffered from headaches at the temple and occasionally saw "flashing lights." His face was very red. His pulse was rapid, wiry and slippery.

DIAGNOSIS

The deep red color shows that there is severe heat. Since the sides are redder and slightly swollen, it is clear that the heat is in the Liver (Liver fire). This is confirmed by the pulse (wiry and rapid) and some of the other symptoms (temporal headache, hypochondriac pain, red face, seeing flashing lights, dream-disturbed sleep). The swelling anteriorly indicates retention of phlegm in the Lungs, the phlegm being caused by deficiency of Spleen qi. This was obviously also the cause of the retention of fluid in the abdomen two years previously, and is confirmed by the slippery pulse.

The coating is particularly interesting: this is one of those rare cases in which a white coating signifies heat. In fact, a white coating like powder denotes heat in the Triple Burner. Furthermore, this coating is rootless, i.e., it is like a powder sprinkled on top of the tongue body rather than growing out of it. This indicates that the Stomach yin has been deficient for a long time. The dryness of the coating is caused by the heat drying up the body fluids.

In conclusion, this patient's asthma was caused by retention of phlegm in the Lungs and also by Liver fire encroaching on the Lungs and stagnating in the chest ("wood insulting metal" from a five-phase perspective). This is a comparatively rare case of asthma attributable to the Liver channel.

PLATE 24: Man, Age 36

TONGUE SIGNS

Body color: deep red
Body shape: deep central crack extending to the tip, many other cracks radiating outward from it; swollen along central crack
Coating: peeled

CASE HISTORY

This patient's main presenting symptom at the time of examination was a kidney-stone lodged in the left ureter. He had stabbing, paroxysmic pain in the left groin. The urine was scanty and very dark. He also had a dry mouth and sweated at night. In the past he had intermittently suffered from asthma from the age of 14 to 34. The pulse was wiry, primarily on the left side, and both proximal positions were weak.

DIAGNOSIS

This tongue clearly shows severe deficiency of Kidney yin, as the color is deep red, there is no coating and there is a very deep crack with several small cracks around it. From this tongue one can diagnose Kidney yin deficiency, rather than just Stomach yin deficiency, because of its deep red color and the very deep central crack extending the entire length of the tongue. In addition, the Kidney yin deficiency has affected the Heart: in fact, deficient Kidney yin failed to nourish Heart yin and this has given rise to deficiency heat in the Heart. This is evidenced by the swelling along the central crack.

PLATE 25: Man, Age 61

TONGUE SIGNS

Body color: normal
Body shape: wide crack in the center that does not extend to the tip; slight cracks on the sides
Coating: no coating

CASE HISTORY

This patient suffered from chronic headaches localized on the forehead, digestive troubles and hemorrhoids. His pulse was weak.

DIAGNOSIS

This tongue is a typical example of Stomach yin deficiency, clearly shown by the wide crack in the center not extending to the tip, and the absence of coating.

The crack deserves more comment: this is a very good example of a central crack related to Stomach yin deficiency because it is wide and shallow and does not reach the tip. (If it were deep and narrow and reached the tip it would indicate a constitutional weakness of the heart.) The slight cracks on the sides of the tongue denote a chronic deficiency of Spleen qi. The whole digestive system, therefore, including the Stomach and Spleen, has been deficient for a long time, causing all his symptoms. The headaches on the forehead are related to the Stomach deficiency. The hemorrhoids are related to the deficiency of Spleen qi.

PLATE 26: Woman, Age 78

TONGUE SIGNS

Body color: red, tip redder
Body shape: crack in the center reaching the tip, other small cracks
Coating: peeled, tip dry, root wet

CASE HISTORY

This patient suffered from deafness for several years and constipation. Her history included pulmonary tuberculosis and a mastectomy to remove a carcinoma of the breast. She also complained of dry eyes. The pulse was floating, empty and slightly rapid.

DIAGNOSIS

The red color and the absence of coating show a deficiency of Kidney yin, which is also reflected in the cracks. Her symptoms, both past and present, point to deficiency of Kidney yin (deafness, constipation and pulmonary tuberculosis). The floating, empty and rapid pulse is also typical of Kidney yin deficiency. The central crack extending to the tip clearly indicates a weakness of the Heart. Because the tip is redder than the body and dry, it also indicates deficiency of the Heart yin. This tongue, therefore, shows a marked pathology of the Kidneys and Heart, which is confirmed by the imbalance of fluids between the root and tip. The root is wet and the tip is dry: this shows an imbalance in the movement of fluids between the Kidneys and Heart. The Kidneys and Heart are not communicating because the Kidney yin is deficient, leading to Heart yin deficiency with resulting deficiency heat of the Heart. The traditional name for this condition is disharmony between the Kidneys and Heart. The dry eyes are also a symptom of the Kidney yin deficiency.

PLATE 27: Woman, Age 63

TONGUE SIGNS

Body color: reddish purple
Body shape: slightly swollen, crack in the center extending to the tip, slightly stiff
Coating: yellow on root, thin and rootless elsewhere, yellow prickles inside the
   crack, generally dry

CASE HISTORY

This patient suffered from chronic rheumatoid arthritis and psoriasis for the past eighteen years. She also had a duodenal ulcer, diagnosed the previous year. The pulse was rapid, full and slippery.

DIAGNOSIS

The reddish purple color and the swelling indicate heat with blood stasis. This was the cause of the psoriasis. A reddish purple and swollen tongue often reflect alcoholism. (This was not the case here, although the patient did consume whiskey and wine every day, which was obviously excessive for her.) The deep crack in the center extending to the tip indicates not only a constitutional weakness of the heart, but also the presence of Heart fire because the tongue body is red. The yellow prickles inside the crack reflect the presence of phlegm-fire in the Stomach and, because they are in the central crack, may also indicate a tendency to mental illness (i.e., "phlegm-fire misting the spirit").

PLATE 28: Woman, Age 93

TONGUE SIGNS

Body color: red
Body shape: normal
Coating: thick, yellow, black and dry, with scattered white, moldy coating on the left side

CASE HISTORY

This patient suffered from lower back pain and some indigestion, with acid regurgitation and constipation.

DIAGNOSIS

The red color of the tongue indicates heat. The thick, yellow, black and dry coating definitely indicates heat in the Stomach and Intestines, with dried-up feces in the Intestines. The scattered, white moldy coating on the left side also reflects heat in the Stomach, which is evaporating its fluids. Because the moldy coating is on the left side, it may suggest that there is also heat in the Liver. The symptoms of indigestion and constipation are due to heat in the Stomach and Intestines. Although this tongue may look quite bad, considering the age of the patient it is actually quite a good tongue. It is not too red, it still has spirit and the problem is mostly confined to the Stomach and Intestines. This lady is, in fact, a very youthful and active 93 years-old.

PLATE 29: Man, Age 46

TONGUE SIGNS

Body color: normal
Body shape: central crack, cracks on the sides, other scattered cracks
Coating: no coating

CASE HISTORY

This patient suffered from migraine headaches at the temple and over the eye-brows. The attacks were accompanied by blurred vision, nausea and dizziness. He also suffered from insomnia. The pulse was leathery, i.e., stretched and tight on the superficial level, and empty on the deep level. This pulse indicates defi-ciency of yin or Kidney essence.

DIAGNOSIS

The absence of coating and the cracks clearly indicate deficiency of Stomach yin. The cracks on the sides denote chronic deficiency of Spleen qi. In this case there is a slight deficiency of Kidney yin not yet manifested on the tongue. The deficiency of Kidney yin induces rising of Liver yang, which accounts for the headaches. The deficiency of Kidney yin is not yet severe enough to give rise to a red tongue. The headaches, in fact, were only of eighteen months' duration.

PLATE 30: Woman, Age 53

TONGUE SIGNS

Body color: bluish purple
Body shape: slightly swollen, crack in the center
Coating: thin and white

CASE HISTORY

This patient suffered from chronic headaches with dull aching on the fore-head and vertex. She also suffered from loose stools and abdominal pain. The pulse was deep, slightly slippery and weak, particularly in both proximal positions.

DIAGNOSIS

The bluish purple tongue body definitely indicates blood stasis due to inter-nal cold. The central crack corresponds to the Stomach and therefore reflects Stomach qi deficiency. The swelling of the tongue body is due to retention of damp-cold resulting from chronic deficiency of Spleen yang and Kidney yang. This is confirmed by the deep and weak pulse on both proximal positions. In sum, the headaches can be attributed to deficiency of Stomach qi, while the loose stools and abdominal pain are caused by the retention of damp-cold in the interior.

PLATE 31: Man, Age 65

TONGUE SIGNS

Body color: reddish purple, tip red
Body shape: swollen (especially on the tip) and stiff
Coating: thin and white, without root, small peeled patches on the root

CASE HISTORY

This patient had suffered a minor stroke, a transient ischemic attack, which left no permanent paralysis. From the perspective of Chinese medicine, this would indicate an attack of internal wind affecting the channels only (not the Organs).

DIAGNOSIS

The reddish purple tongue body indicates heat with blood stasis. The red tip indicates Heart fire. The swelling of the body is, in this case, due to heat. The stiff body denotes the presence of internal wind, in this case stirred by the interior heat. One can therefore deduce that the heat is in the Liver and has given rise to wind, and that the Liver blood is stagnant. The Heart fire probably also derives from the Liver fire. The rootless coating and the peeled patches on the root reflect yin deficiency of the Stomach affecting the Intestines.

In sum, this tongue reflects a chronic condition and presents three of the four conditions predisposing to wind-stroke: internal wind, fire and stagnation (the fourth being phlegm).

PLATE 32: Woman, Age 29

TONGUE SIGNS

Body color: normal
Body shape: normal, except for a swelling superficially on the right half
Coating: normal

CASE HISTORY

This patient had suffered a collapsed lung two years previously.

DIAGNOSIS

This tongue is included primarily to illustrate the swelling on half the surface of the tongue on the right side. This swelling is of a deficient nature and is due to the collapse of the right lung.

PLATE 33: Man, Age 30

TONGUE SIGNS

Body color: normal except for a slightly red left side and tip
Body shape: normal, except for very slight swelling on the left side
Coating: yellow and slippery on the left side

CASE HISTORY

This patient had hepatitis two months previously. He also suffered from nervous tension and dream-disturbed sleep. The pulse was full, rapid and slippery.

DIAGNOSIS

All the tongue signs appear on the left side (red body, slight swelling and yellow-slippery coating). This clearly points to a Liver problem. In this case, it indicates retention of damp-heat in the Liver and Gallbladder.

PLATE 34: Woman, Age 54

TONGUE SIGNS

Body color: normal
Body shape: very swollen (especially on the sides), many deep cracks on the sides
Coating: dry, powder-like, rootless

CASE HISTORY

This patient complained of soreness in several different joints and muscles: fingers, hip, knees and upper back. These pains were a form of painful obstruction *(bi)* disorder from damp-cold, but were also affected by the patient's several falls from horses over the years. These falls caused stagnation of qi in the joints and muscles and slowed down the circulation of blood, which contributed to the pain. All of these are channel problems and were not, in this case, reflected on the tongue. However, she also complained of poor digestion, no appetite, loose stools and dull headaches. The pulse was slow and slippery.

DIAGNOSIS

In this case the body shape assumes foremost importance. The grossly swollen tongue body and sides and the very deep cracks on the sides point to a severe and chronic deficiency of Spleen qi which is unable to move fluids (as shown by the dryness of the coating). There is also dampness, reflected in the swelling of the tongue body and the slow and slippery pulse. The powder-like coating is an extreme form of rootless coating which denotes extreme deficiency of Stomach yin.

It is remarkable how the cracks can disappear, as can be seen in the subsequent picture of the same patient's tongue two years later.

PLATE 35: Same As Above, Two Years Later

PLATES 36, 37 & 38: Girl, Age 10

These three photographs show a sequence in the progression and regression of the pathogenic influences in chicken pox in a 10-year-old child.

PLATE 36

TONGUE SIGNS

Body color: normal, with red points all around the tip and sides
Body shape: normal
Coating: yellow and sticky

DIAGNOSIS

This is the first stage in an attack of wind-dampness and heat. The pathogenic influence is in the exterior because the red points are all around the edges and tip; there is dampness because the coating is slippery; and there is heat because the coating is yellow and there are red points. The dampness is also denoted by the pus contained in the pustules, and the heat is further shown by the fact that the pustules have a red edge, are raised and are painful.

PLATE 37

TONGUE SIGNS

Body color: same, red points still there
Body shape: normal
Coating: still yellow, more slippery

DIAGNOSIS

The slippery coating signifies more dampness. This is reflected by the pustules containing more pus and being near to eruption. The differentiation between this stage (when the pustules are breaking) and the previous one (at the onset when the pustules have just appeared and are hard) is all-important in Chinese medicine, as the treatment is different for each stage. In the first stage the therapeutic principle of resolving the fire toxin is applied, and in the latter stage (when the pustules are soft and breaking) the therapeutic principle of resolving phlegm is applied. When Chinese herbs are prescribed, quite different herbs would be used at each stage.

PLATE 38

TONGUE SIGNS

Body color: normal, the red points are now pale red and not so raised
Body shape: normal
Coating: thin and white, not sticky or slippery

DIAGNOSIS

This tongue shows a definite improvement in the condition and a regression of the pathogenic factor. The red points are now pale red and not so raised; this shows that the heat has subsided. The coating is white instead of yellow, and is not sticky; this also shows that the heat has subsided and that the dampness has been resolved.

PLATE 39: Woman, Age 41

TONGUE SIGNS

Body color: red, sides slightly purple
Body shape: normal
Underside: vein on right side purple and distended

CASE HISTORY

This patient suffered from premenstrual tension and experienced irritability, depression and distension of breasts before the onset of her period, which was painful. She had also been suffering from headaches for several years, with pain at the right temple, dizziness and tinnitus. Occasionally she experienced a stabbing pain in the chest. She was constipated and occasionally suffered from cystitis, with frequency and burning on urination. She was also chronically fatigued. The pulse was deep, slightly wiry on the left side and slightly choppy on the right.

DIAGNOSIS

The red tongue body, slightly purple on the sides, indicates blood stasis and heat. The blood stasis is confirmed by the purple color and distension of the right vein on the underside of the tongue. The fact that only the right vein is distended (the left vein is beginning to show distension at the base) indicates that the blood stasis is concentrated more in the channels on the right side of the body. This is probably the cause of the right-sided headaches. Most of her symptoms and signs can be attributed to stasis of Liver blood (premenstrual tension, headache and the stabbing pain in the chest). The dizziness and tinnitus are due to the rising of Liver yang, and the constipation and tendency to cystitis are caused by the downward infusion of Liver fire. The wiry quality of the pulse on the left side indicates stasis of Liver blood, while the choppy quality on the right side indicates deficiency of Stomach and Spleen and a pre-existing condition of blood deficiency. This accounts for the extreme, chronic fatigue.

PLATE 41: Boy , Age 7

TONGUE SIGNS

Body color: red, especially in the front part, red points around the center
Body shape: swollen in the front part
Coating: thick, yellow, with root

CASE HISTORY

This boy had contracted an upper respiratory infection four days prior to examination. His initial symptoms included a sore throat, swollen glands, shivering, fever and body aches. When the photo was taken his symptoms had changed and included cough with expectoration of yellow sputum, fever, a feeling of heat, thirst and restlessness.

DIAGNOSIS

The initial symptoms are typical of an invasion of external wind-heat in the defensive qi portion of the Lungs. When the photo was taken the pathogenic factor had progressed into the interior and affected the Lungs. From the perspective of the four levels identification of patterns, it corresponded to Lung heat at the qi level.

The red tongue body indicates interior heat, and its concentration in the front part confirms its location in the Lungs. The red points around the center are left over from the exterior stage when they would be concentrated on the sides. The swelling in the front part denotes that there is not only Lung heat, but also Lung phlegm-heat. The thick, yellow coating with root confirms the presence of interior heat from excess.

PLATE 42: Boy, Age 9

TONGUE SIGNS

Body color: red, redder in the front part, red points in the center
Body shape: swollen in the front part
Coating: absent from the front part and toward the center, thin, yellow and slightly rootless elsewhere

CASE HISTORY

This patient (the same person as in the previous case) had contracted an acute upper respiratory tract infection eight days prior to examination. His initial symptoms included a sore throat, body aches and fever. He then developed a chest infection with fever, cough with yellow sputum, tonsillitis and a feeling of heat. He was given antibiotics at this stage, and although these helped the chest infection and the cough, his condition did not improve at all. His fever continued (especially in the evening), he still had a feeling of heat, felt thirsty and restless, did not sleep well and his tonsils were still swollen.

DIAGNOSIS

The initial symptoms correspond to an invasion of wind-heat, and the second stage (with the chest infection) is typical of Lung phlegm-heat at the qi level. At the time of examination when the picture was taken, his condition had just begun to enter the nutritive qi level. The red color of the body, together with the absence of coating in the front and center, clearly indicates deficiency heat. This is a definite sign that the condition is at the nutritive qi level. In fact, the tongue is the most reliable indicator for showing the progression from the qi to the nutritive qi level: at the qi level it has a thick yellow coating on a red body (indicating excess heat), and at the nutritive qi level it is darker red and without coating (indicating deficiency heat).

In this case the boy had just entered the nutritive qi level; children can move from one level to the next very quickly. It is important to note that although the signs and symptoms described for the nutritive qi level are very serious, in children these can take a milder form, as is the case here. In children a tongue such as that portrayed in the photo can change back to almost normal within one day, as was the case with this boy.

PLATE 43: Woman, Age 32

TONGUE SIGNS

Body color: pale overall, but red on the root
Body shape: swollen, tooth-marked
Coating: thin, sticky, white overall except on the root, which is peeled

CASE HISTORY

This patient suffered from Addison's disease. Her main signs and symptoms were extreme lassitude, constipation, poor appetite, pigmentation of the skin, dry skin, dry mouth, night sweating and a feeling of heat in the face, which was worse in the evening. Her pulse was weak on both proximal positions.

DIAGNOSIS

The red color and peeling on the root of the tongue clearly shows a deficiency of Kidney yin with deficiency heat. This type of tongue is rather an exception to the normal development of yin deficiency in which, by the time Kidney yin becomes deficient, the whole tongue is usually red and peeled (see chapter 5). In this case, only the root is red and peeled. A possible explanation is the presence of not only Kidney deficiency in a Chinese medical sense, but also an actual kidney pathology from a biomedical perspective (bearing in mind that the cortex of the adrenal glands forms part of the Kidneys). Kidney deficiency is confirmed by the weakness of the pulse at both proximal positions, and by the symptoms of night sweating, dry skin, dry mouth and extreme lassitude.

PLATE 44: Woman, Age 30

TONGUE SIGNS

Body color: normal, red points on front part
Body shape: slightly thin, tooth-marked
Coating: peeled in patches ("geographic" tongue)

CASE HISTORY

This patient suffered from sarcoidosis of the lungs. The main clinical manifestations were: a dry cough, breathlessness, wheezing, a dry throat and night sweating. Her pulse was floating-empty.

DIAGNOSIS

All her symptoms and signs are very typical of Lung yin deficiency: dry cough, dry throat, breathlessness and night sweating. The floating-empty quality of the pulse is also indicative of yin deficiency.

The tooth-marked tongue indicates Spleen qi deficiency, while the coating peeled in patches indicates Stomach yin deficiency. Thus, the tongue clearly reflects two patterns (Spleen qi deficiency and Stomach yin deficiency) which are not apparent from the symptoms, but are nevertheless closely linked with the pathology of this case. In fact, both the Spleen and Stomach are the "mother" of the Lungs from a five-phase perspective, and their deficiency is often the basis of a Lung deficiency disorder. Stomach yin deficiency, in particular, is often the basis of Lung yin deficiency.

PLATE 45: Man, Age 45

TONGUE SIGNS

Body color: pale
Body shape: swollen, tooth-marked, Stomach-Heart crack
Coating: sticky-white coating overall, slightly yellow in the center toward the root

CASE HISTORY

This patient had suffered from extreme anxiety for many years. He had been put on tranquillizers 15 years previously and developed an addiction to them. His symptoms worsened and he resorted to higher and higher doses of tranquillizers. He was finally taken off of them and suffered a complete nervous breakdown. After that he resumed taking tranquillizers, albeit in a smaller dose, and at this point came for a consultation.

This man suffered from very severe anxiety manifesting with palpitations, sweating and tremors. He did not sleep well and his bowels were always loose, with several movements in the morning. A peculiar feature of his anxiety was that it worsened (he "fell to pieces") whenever his sister, who lived in the same town, went on holiday.

DIAGNOSIS

The very swollen tongue body and sticky coating are clear signs of phlegm. The paleness of the body and tooth-marks indicate Spleen qi deficiency, which is obviously at the base of phlegm. His severe anxiety is caused by phlegm obstructing and harassing the spirit.

PLATE 46: Woman, Age 53

TONGUE SIGNS

Body color: pale
Body shape: swollen, more so in the front part, tooth-marked
Coating: sticky white all over

CASE HISTORY

This patient suffered from what was diagnosed as manic-depression. During the depressive phase she would feel very depressed and tired, while during the manic phase she would engage in frenetic and chaotic activity, without bringing anything to completion. On the whole she felt cold and tired, and her stools were loose.

DIAGNOSIS

This is a case of the spirit being obstructed by phlegm. The swollen tongue body and sticky coating clearly denote phlegm. The pale color of the tongue body and tooth marks indicate Spleen qi deficiency, which is the basis for the formation of phlegm. Her fatigue, loose stools and cold feeling are also indicative of Spleen qi deficiency.

PLATE 47: Man, Age 28

TONGUE SIGNS

Body color: red, tip redder and with red points
Body shape: slightly stiff
Coating: thick, yellow, dry coating
Moisture: very dry

CASE HISTORY

This patient complained of insomnia, anxiety and a feeling of heat. On questioning, it transpired that he also suffered from constipation, thirst and palpitations. His pulse was full and slightly overflowing at the left distal position.

DIAGNOSIS

This tongue is a classic example of excess heat: it is red, has a yellow coating with root, and is very dry. The redder tip with red points clearly locates the excess heat in the Heart. The thick, yellow and dry coating (together with the symptom of constipation) signifies the presence of heat in the Stomach and Intestines, as the coating reflects the state of the yang more than the yin organs. The slight stiffness of the tongue body indicates that the heat is beginning to injure the body fluids, which is confirmed by its dryness.

The symptoms of palpitations, anxiety, insomnia and a feeling of heat clearly confirm the presence of Heart fire.

A tongue such as this, with a bright red tip with red points, is a strong indication that emotional stress is at the root of the condition, which was in fact the case here.

PLATE 48: Woman, Age 72

TONGUE SIGNS

Body color: red
Body shape: slightly thin, although the sides are slightly swollen, scattered cracks
Coating: peeled, except for a very small area toward the root

CASE HISTORY

This patient complained of Meniere's syndrome: she had been suffering from severe vertigo, nausea, and tinnitus for the past ten years. She also complained of loose stools with abdominal pain and distension, lower backache and night sweating. Her pulse was thin in general, weaker on the right side, and slightly wiry on the left.

DIAGNOSIS

The red color of the tongue body, together with the lack of coating, clearly indicates yin deficiency with deficiency heat. The symptoms of backache, tinnitus and night sweating denote that Kidney yin is deficient. The severe vertigo and nausea are caused by the rising of Liver yang, itself caused by the deficiency of Kidney yin.

One positive aspect of this tongue is that it is *not* dry: this is favorable sign because it shows that the deficient yin has not yet affected the body fluids. The thin tongue body confirms the deficiency of yin. The slight swelling of the sides denotes Spleen deficiency; this is its only sign on the tongue. The symptom of loose stools confirms this. The abdominal pain and distension is due to stagnant Liver qi invading the Spleen. (This last pattern can only be deduced from the symptoms and pulse, not from the tongue.)

PLATE 49: Woman, Age 54

TONGUE SIGNS

Body color: reddish purple, red points in the front part
Body shape: swollen, Heart crack, tooth-marked
Coating: generally sticky white, sticky yellow inside the crack toward the root (yellow prickles), peeled in patches, especially on the sides toward the front (chest area)

CASE HISTORY

This patient had been suffering from angina pectoris for several years. Her main signs and symptoms included: a feeling of oppression of the chest, a stabbing pain in the chest, cough with yellow sputum, insomnia, night sweating, a feeling of heat in the evening, tiredness and epigastric distension and fullness. Her pulse was slippery on the whole, but also empty on the deep level, especially on the left side.

DIAGNOSIS

This is a very complex case with an intricate pathology. The tongue itself shows all the aspects of the condition. First of all, the reddish purple body indicates heat with stasis of blood. The redness and peeling on the front part of the tongue (chest area) indicate that the heat and the stasis of blood occur mostly in the chest; thus, there is Lung deficiency heat and stasis of blood in the chest. The red points in this area indicate the severity of the Lung deficiency heat. The peeled patches indicate deficiency of Stomach yin, while the stickiness of the coating and the swelling of the tongue body denote the presence of phlegm. The yellow prickles inside the Heart crack indicate that phlegm-heat is affecting the Heart. The tooth marks indicate Spleen qi deficiency, which is the basis for the formation of phlegm.

This tongue thus shows a complex combination of deficiency and excess: there is deficiency of Spleen qi, Stomach yin and Lung yin, and excess of phlegm-heat, deficiency heat, and stasis of blood.

As for the symptoms, phlegm is indicated by the feeling of oppression in the chest, cough with yellow sputum and epigastric distension and fullness. The pain in the chest denotes stasis of blood; insomnia, night sweating and feeling of heat in the evening are indicative of deficiency heat, while tiredness is due to Spleen qi deficiency.

PLATE 50: Woman, Age 53

TONGUE SIGNS

Body color: slightly pale, especially on the sides
Body shape: slightly swollen overall, much more so in the front part; slightly tooth-marked
Coating: normal, slightly sticky

CASE HISTORY

This patient suffered from late-onset asthma. This is asthma which starts in middle age and is not associated with eczema. As such it is contrasted with early-onset asthma, which starts during early childhood and is usually associated with atopic eczema. This patient was often wheezy and had to resort to a nonsteroidal inhaler (Ventolin) about three times a day. She also had a feeling of oppression in the chest and epigastrium, and felt very tired. Her body felt heavy and her chest was obstructed by catarrh. Her pulse was slippery on the whole, but weak on the right side.

DIAGNOSIS

The tongue very clearly shows the presence of phlegm (swollen with a slightly sticky coating); the obvious swelling in the front part shows that the phlegm is obstructing the Lungs. The tooth marks indicate Spleen qi deficiency, which is the basis for the formation of phlegm. Her other symptoms clearly point to the presence of phlegm: feeling of oppression and heaviness, catarrh in the chest and wheezing. The tiredness is due both to phlegm itself and to the deficiency of the Spleen.

PLATE 51: Man, Age 45

TONGUE SIGNS

Body color: normal
Body shape: deviated, swollen, deep Heart crack
Coating: sticky white, except in the crack where it is yellow

CASE HISTORY

This patient had suffered a stroke (cerebral thrombosis) six months previously. This left him with hemiplegia and numbness of the limbs on the affected side. His speech was slightly slurred and he felt very tired. Other manifestations included blurred vision, cramps in the legs at night and a pulse which was empty at the deep level.

DIAGNOSIS

The tongue actually shows two of the pathogenic elements which led to the wind-stroke. The clear deviation indicates Liver wind, while the swelling of the tongue body and the sticky coating denote phlegm: wind and phlegm are the two major pathogenic factors which lead to stroke. There must also obviously be some Spleen qi deficiency, which leads to the formation of phlegm, and Liver blood or Liver yin deficiency, leads to Liver wind. However, these two deficiencies are not showing on the tongue. The blurred vision, leg cramps and pulse (empty at the deep level) indicate Liver yin deficiency, while tiredness indicates Spleen qi deficiency.

PLATE 52: Man, Age 37

TONGUE SIGNS

Body color: normal
Body shape: deep scattered cracks, swollen, a few transverse Spleen cracks on the edges
Coating: no coating

CASE HISTORY

This patient suffered from AIDS. He had been largely symptom-free for three years from the time he was diagnosed as being HIV-positive. In recent months, however, he had been suffering from recurrent low-grade fevers and infections. He felt hot, sweated at night, and had a dry cough and throat. His bowels were loose, his appetite was poor and he felt very tired. His pulse was generally floating and empty.

DIAGNOSIS

The tongue shows a very clear deficiency of Stomach yin, being completely peeled. The deep, scattered cracks confirm the severity of the deficiency of Stomach yin. The few transverse cracks on the edges also point to Spleen yin deficiency. The swelling of the tongue body indicates dampness or phlegm, which derives from Spleen qi deficiency. His symptoms, however, also show Lung yin deficiency (dry throat and cough). Other general symptoms of yin deficiency include the feeling of heat, night sweats and the floating and empty pulse. The loose bowels, poor appetite and tiredness indicates Spleen qi deficiency.

PLATE 53: Same Patient as PLATE 52

TONGUE SIGNS

Body color: red, especially in the front part
Body shape: swollen, deep cracks
Coating: thick, sticky yellow coating, without root in the front part

CASE HISTORY

This photo was taken three days after PLATE 52, during an acute episode of pneumonia.

DIAGNOSIS

The body shape is the same: it is still swollen and there are obviously the same cracks. The body color has become red, indicating the presence of interior heat. The sudden appearance of the thick yellow coating clearly indicates a worsening of the condition and is due to the development of intense, interior Lung phlegm-heat; the concentration of this coating in the front part clearly relates to the Lungs. However, this coating is without root, as the tongue was previously peeled. The fact that the coating appeared suddenly and is thick, yellow and rootless definitely indicates a worsening of the condition. It would be a great mistake to interpret the appearance of this coating on a previously peeled tongue as a favorable sign (see chapter 7).

PLATE 54: Same Patient as PLATES 52 & 53

TONGUE SIGNS

Body color: normal to red, white vesicles in the front

Body shape: swollen, deep cracks
Coating: no coating, except for scattered patches of rootless coating

CASE HISTORY

This photo was taken four days after PLATE 53. At this time, the patient had recovered from pneumonia and his fever had abated.

DIAGNOSIS

The tongue reverted to its original state in that it is no longer red. There are, however, some new signs. The white vesicles in the front indicate retention of dampness in the Lungs, obviously left over from the phlegm-heat. The scattered patches of rootless coating are also left over from the previous thick yellow coating found in the acute stage; these indicate the retention of a residual pathogenic factor.

PLATE 55: Man, Age 75

TONGUE SIGNS

Body color: red, yellowish veins underside, with purple venules
Body shape: thin
Coating: no coating

CASE HISTORY

This man suffered from chronic angina pectoris. His signs and symptoms included a feeling of oppression and pain in the chest, breathlessness on exertion, a feeling of heat, thirst and a wiry pulse.

DIAGNOSIS

The underside of the tongue shows that the body is red: this indicates heat. The veins themselves indicate dampness steaming upwards in the upper burner, while the purple venules indicate stasis of blood. Thus, this man's condition, called chest painful obstruction in Chinese medicine, is clearly due to obstruction of the chest qi by phlegm and stasis of blood.

PLATE 56: Woman, Age 28

TONGUE SIGNS

Body color: pale, wet
Body shape: slightly swollen
Coating: no coating

CASE HISTORY

This patient suffered from exhaustion, her principal complaint. Upon inquiring it transpired that her periods were very scanty, lasting only one day. She was also often dizzy and her vision was blurred at times. Her appetite was poor, her stools were usually loose and she always felt cold. Her pulse was weak on the right and thin on the left.

DIAGNOSIS

The pale and peeled tongue (like a 'plucked chicken') is a clear sign of severe blood deficiency, which was confirmed by the scanty periods, exhaustion, dizziness, blurred vision and thin pulse. The wetness of the tongue contradicts this diagnosis inasmuch as the tongue should be dry where there is blood deficiency. However, the tongue is wet here because she also has Spleen yang deficiency; this is confirmed by the cold feeling, loose stools, lack of appetite and weak pulse.

PLATE 57: Woman, Age 38

TONGUE SIGNS

Body color: normal, red on the root, slightly dry
Body shape: slightly swollen, especially in the front part, transverse Spleen cracks on the edges
Coating: peeled in patches ("geographic"), none on the root

CASE HISTORY

This patient suffered from migraine and digestive disorders. Her migraine was characterized by a throbbing pain on the temples and was accompanied by some dizziness and nausea. Her digestion was poor. She suffered from constipation (with normal-sized stools) and abdominal pain and distension.

DIAGNOSIS

This is a complex condition in that the tongue signs and clinical manifestations each point to different aspects of the disorder. The tongue itself shows yin deficiency of the Stomach and Kidneys: the peeling of the tongue in patches indicates Stomach yin deficiency, while the peeling of the root denotes Kidney yin deficiency. The transverse cracks on the edges indicate that there is also Spleen yin deficiency, while the swelling denotes Spleen qi deficiency.

The symptoms indicate Liver yang rising (migraine headaches of the throbbing type on the temples, with dizziness and nausea) and some Liver qi stagnation (abdominal pain and distension). The constipation is due to yin deficiency; it may have also been due to Liver qi stagnation, but this is not the case as the stools themselves are not small.

PLATE 58: Same Patient as PLATE 57

TONGUE SIGNS

Body color: normal, slightly red on the root
Body shape: slightly swollen, transverse Spleen cracks on the edges
Coating: peeled in patches

CASE HISTORY

See PLATE 57 above.

DIAGNOSIS

This photo, taken three months after the previous one, shows an improvement in the woman's condition. The color of the root is less red, the tongue body is less dry, the Spleen cracks are less deep and, most importantly, some coating has returned on the root. All of this indicates that the deficiency of yin is less severe.

PLATE 59: Man, Age 72

TONGUE SIGNS

Body color: reddish purple, dry
Body shape: swollen, long, deep, scattered cracks
Coating: none except for some patches of thick, yellow, rootless coating

CASE HISTORY

This patient had been suffering from late-onset asthma and bronchitis for several years. He was often wheezy and breathless and suffered from a chronic cough productive of scanty, tenacious, yellow sputum. He also suffered from lower backache, dizziness, tinnitus, night sweats and a dry throat at night. His pulse was rapid, floating and empty.

DIAGNOSIS

The tongue shows a very severe yin deficiency of the Stomach, Kidneys, and Lungs. The yin deficiency of the Stomach and Kidneys is evident from the red and peeled tongue body, while that of the Lungs is denoted by the large, deep cracks, which tend to be in the front part (Lung area). This finding is confirmed by the dry throat at night and the chronic cough. The latter symptom is indicative of both yin deficiency and phlegm: the scanty, tenacious sputum denotes dry phlegm. This is old, chronic phlegm which becomes dry and is only seen among the elderly with yin deficiency and phlegm.

The symptoms of backache, dizziness, tinnitus, night sweating and a floating, empty pulse clearly indicate Kidney yin deficiency.

The purple color of the tongue body indicates stasis of blood. This is probably located in the chest due to the chronic retention of phlegm obstructing the circulation of qi and blood in that region.

The thick yellow coating indicates phlegm-heat, while its rootlessness signifies that there is an underlying yin deficiency. A thick coating without root represents the "worst of both worlds," as the absence of root indicates yin deficiency, while thickness denotes the presence of a strong pathogenic factor; there is thus simultaneous excess and deficiency.

Appendices

I
Identification of Patterns According to the Six Stages

INTRODUCTION

The identification of patterns according to the six stages is one of the most important theoretical frameworks in traditional Chinese clinical diagnosis and treatment. The bulk of this theory was formulated by the famous physician Zhang Zhong-Jing in his book, *Discussion of Cold-induced Disorders* (c. 220). While on one level this book may be said to focus on the symptomatology and treatment of diseases caused by external cold alone, it is in fact a cornerstone of Chinese medicine's clinical symptomatology and treatment of both exterior and interior diseases from cold or heat.

Zhang Zhong-Jing was born during the Han dynasty between 158 and 166 A.D. His original work on diseases derived from cold was published in sixteen volumes, later divided into two parts: *Discussion of Cold-induced Disorders* and *Essentials of the Golden Cabinet*. Portions of his original work, first edited by Wang Shu-He, the famous sphygmologist of the Jin dynasty, were subsequently lost. The edition currently used dates from the Song dynasty (960-1279).

The *Discussion of Cold-induced Disorders* provides the theoretical framework for the diagnosis and treatment of diseases caused by externally-contracted cold, generally manifesting with fever. In the preface to this work, Zhang said that of the roughly 200 inhabitants of his village, more than two-thirds had died within the previous ten years. Seventy percent of these had died of enteric fevers. Zhang's great work stems from an era when epidemics and various types of enteric fevers were the most prevalent disorders. However, the symptomatology of the *Discussion of Cold-induced Disorders* is also applicable to our times and conditions. It describes the essential features and patterns of several types of fevers, and of externally-contracted diseases in general.

The clinical manifestations of diseases contracted from attack by external cold are arranged by Zhang according to six stages, corresponding to the six channels: greater yang (Small Intestine and Bladder); yang brightness (Large Intestine and Stomach); lesser yang (Triple Burner and Gallbladder); greater yin (Lungs and Spleen); lesser yin (Heart and Kidneys); and terminal yin (Pericardium and Liver). Only the greater yang stage reflects an exterior condition (cold). All of the other stages are interior conditions.

Essential to an understanding of the progression of disease through these stages is the concept of struggle between the external pathogenic factor and the body's qi. Most of the clinical manifestations are due to this struggle and the constantly changing strength of these two forces relative to each other. It is also the relative strength or weakness of the pathogenic factor and of the body's qi that determines whether the pattern is one of deficiency or excess.

A pattern of excess is characterized by a strong pathogenic factor, but also by relatively strong qi. The struggle between these two forces causes the rather violent symptoms typical of a pattern of excess. A pattern of deficiency, on the other hand, is characterized by the continued presence of a pathogenic factor and weakness of the body's qi, which is not reacting to that factor. The symptoms associated with a pattern of deficiency are of a more subdued nature than those of a pattern of excess.

Another important concept in this diagnostic system is that of depth of the disease. One of the primary aims of this system of differentiation is to provide a framework within which the depth of a disease can be determined. In the three yang stages the disease is more superficial and affects the yang channels or yang Organs. In the three yin stages the disease is deeper and affects the yin Organs. Just as the clinical manifestations vary according to the relative strength or weakness of the pathogenic factor and the body's qi, they also vary according to the depth of the disease. In the three yang stages the pathogenic factor is predominant, the body's qi is still relatively strong, there are signs of excess heat and treatment is directed at eliminating the pathogenic factor. In the three yin stages the pathogenic factor is still present but is diminishing, the body's qi has been weakened, there are signs of cold from deficiency and treatment is focused upon strengthening the body's qi.

This intricate and detailed evaluation of complex clinical signs is one of the best features of Chinese medicine. It permits the identification of the predominant pattern and thus the appropriate treatment for a particular condition at a particular point in its evolution.

In the discussion below, the biomedical pathological conditions overlapping each traditional Chinese pattern will be identified whenever possible. Bear in spirit, however, that there is no direct correspondence between biomedically-defined diseases and Chinese disorders. For example, the onset of a common cold could correspond to the greater yang stage of the six stages, or to the defensive-qi level of the four levels, or to the upper burner stage of the three burners. In the same manner, the greater yang stage could correspond to the onset of a multitude of different biomedically-defined diseases. These correspondences are discussed only when they are useful in clinical practice.

GREATER YANG

The greater yang stage corresponds to the onset of a disease from attack by external cold. From the perspective of the eight principles, it is a stage of exterior excess cold. The key clinical manifestations are aversion to cold, shivers, fever, a stiff neck, headache and a floating pulse.

The greater yang channels (corresponding to the Small Intestine and Bladder) govern the exterior of the body. These are the most superficial channels, rich in supply of defensive qi, whose function is to resist invasion by external pathogenic factors. When wind-cold invades the body the greater yang channels are the first to be affected. The invasion of external wind-cold hinders the circulation of defensive qi. This results in pain and stiffness of the head and neck (at the occiput) where the greater yang channels flow.

The struggle between the exterior wind-cold and the defensive qi results in fever. The presence of wind-cold in the muscles results in aversion to cold. As the exterior wind-cold invades the defensive qi portion of the body, both defensive and nutritive qi surge outward to oppose the external pathogenic factor. The whole body's energy moves toward the surface, resulting in a floating pulse. The tongue body color is unchanged because the disease only affects the exterior. There may be a thin, white coating more on the front or the sides of the tongue, reflecting the exterior location of the disease. The white color of the coating signifies the cold nature of the pathogenic factor.

This description of clinical manifestations in external attacks of wind-cold is very generalized. In practice it is important to distinguish between attacks of cold and attacks of wind since the treatment in each case will differ, even though, e.g., the rationale for the occurrence of fever and pain or stiffness in the head and neck applies to both conditions.

Attack of Wind

When wind predominates over cold, clinical symptoms will include fever, sweating, slight shivers, aversion to wind, pain and stiffness in the head and neck and a floating, slow pulse.

This pattern is characterized by relative weakness of the nutritive qi compared to the defensive qi. The sweating is caused by the weakness of the nutritive qi, which makes the pores flaccid. However, there is only slight — not profuse — sweating. The failure of the defensive qi to warm the skin and muscles results in aversion to wind. Aversion to wind and aversion to cold are basically similar in nature; they only differ in intensity. Aversion to wind is less intense than aversion to cold and only occurs when a person is outdoors. Aversion to cold is stronger and can occur even if a person is indoors.

The pulse is floating because the body's qi surges outward to meet the patho-genic wind. The pulse is also slow because the body's qi is relatively weak.

From a biomedical perspective, diseases including the common cold and other upper respiratory tract infections may present with this pattern.

Attack of Cold

When cold predominates over wind, clinical manifestations will include fever, absence of sweating, aversion to cold, pronounced shivers, pain and stiffness in the head and neck, generalized aching of the body, lower back pain, shortness of breath and a floating, tight pulse.

Generalized body aches and lower back pain are caused by the external cold's obstruction of the circulation of defensive qi in the skin and muscles. In particu-lar, lower back pain is caused by stagnation of qi in the greater yang channel of the lower back. Cold contracts; hence, the pores are contracted and there is no sweating. The contraction caused by cold impairs the Lungs' dispersing and descending functions and leads to shortness of breath. The pulse is floating because the body's qi surges outward to meet the pathogenic cold; it is tight because of the contracting nature of cold.

Cold in the exterior, closure of pores and impairment of the Lungs' dispers-ing and descending functions may be treated by releasing the exterior, opening the pores to cause sweating and promoting the Lungs' dispersing and descending functions. The treatment for an attack of cold is more vigorous than that for an attack of wind. The latter should be milder because of the sweating and the rela-tive deficiency of nutritive qi. In other words, although attacks of wind and cold are both patterns of excess, an attack of wind is also a partially deficient pattern due to the relative deficiency of nutritive qi. In actual practice, for attacks of cold it is essential to cause sweating and to apply a strong treatment, e.g., a reducing technique when acupuncture is utilized. For attacks of wind, a milder form of treatment should be chosen.

When we contrast attacks of wind and attacks of cold we find that sweating occurs in attacks of wind, but not in attacks of cold. The pulse is slow and floating in attacks of wind, and tight and floating in attacks of cold. In the latter there is shortness of breath and general body aches, symptoms which are absent in attacks of wind.

From a biomedical perspective, diseases including the common cold, influenza and pneumonia may present with this pattern.

YANG BRIGHTNESS

The yang brightness stage develops from the greater yang or lesser yang stages of an externally-contracted disorder due to an attack of cold. It is characterized by penetration of the pathogenic factor to the interior, specifically to the Stomach and Large Intestine (yang brightness) channels and Organs. This stage is also characterized by the relative strength of both the pathogenic factor and the body's energies. This results in a pattern of excess. Furthermore, in the yang brightness stage the pathogenic factor has transformed into heat.

Although this stage is traditionally studied in the context of the six-stage identification of patterns from attack of cold, it is a common interior pattern. Whether or not it is caused by external cold is irrelevant; the clinical manifestations can be interpreted according to Zhang's analysis and treated accordingly.

Within the yang brightness stage there are two variations: pure interior heat (yang brightness channel stage), and interior heat with constipation (yang brightness Organ stage).

Yang Brightness Channel Stage

The yang brightness channel stage affects the yang brightness channels but not the Organs themselves. Clinical manifestations include high fever, profuse sweating, thirst, a strong desire to drink cold water, redness of the face, restlessness, a red tongue body, a yellow, thick, dry tongue coating and a big, overflowing pulse.

The high fever is a reflection of the intense struggle between the pathogenic factor and the body's energies. The red face and restlessness are symptoms of heat. The sweating is due to interior heat dispersing the body fluids outward. The thirst and dry tongue coating are a reflection of the desiccation of the body's fluids caused by interior heat. In this case thirst is a very prominent symptom and the patient definitely prefers to drink large amounts of cold water. The overflowing pulse reflects the relative strength of the body's qi and of the pathogenic factor, as well as the presence of heat. It is important to note that if the patient is sweating profusely, heat signs may be less obvious since heat is dispersed by the sweating. The signs of this stage are often referred to as the "four bigs," consisting of big (high) fever, big (severe) thirst, big (profuse) sweating and a big (or overflowing) pulse.

From a biomedical perspective, diseases including influenza, pneumonia and encephalitis B may present with this pattern.

Yang Brightness Organ Stage

The yang brightness Organ stage affects the Stomach and Large Intestine. Clinical signs include fever that is worse in the afternoon, constipation, fullness and pain in the abdomen that becomes worse with pressure, restlessness and irritability, a red tongue body, a yellow, thick, dry tongue coating, or a brown or black coating with prickles, and a deep, full pulse. In severe cases, there may also be delirium.

The fever associated with this stage is again caused by the struggle between a pathogenic factor and the body's qi. The fever is higher in the afternoon but is present throughout the day. This is in contrast to yin-deficiency fever, which tends to be present only in the afternoon and evening. The constipation and feeling of fullness and pain in the abdomen are due to pathogenic heat having dried up the body fluids. There are desiccated feces in the Intestines obstructing the free circulation of qi, which itself aggravates the pain. The irritability, restlessness and delirium are caused by the disturbance of the spirit by interior heat. The dry tongue coating reflects the consumption of body fluids by heat, and the deep pulse indicates the obstruction of the interior by desiccated feces. The tongue coating in this stage is thicker than in the yang brightness channel stage.

When we compare the yang brightness channel and Organ stages we find that both are characterized by interior excess heat with fever, thirst and a yellow, dry tongue coating. When we contrast these stages we see that in the channel stage there is profuse sweating and a big pulse. In the Organ stage there is constipation, fullness and pain in the abdomen and a deep pulse. The channel stage is treated by clearing the heat, and the Organ stage both by clearing the heat and relieving the constipation.

From a biomedical perspective, diseases including influenza, pneumonia and enteritis may present with this pattern.

LESSER YANG

The lesser yang stage usually progresses from the greater yang stage and is characterized by invasion of the Gallbladder channel by a pathogenic factor (usually heat, transformed from cold). Greater yang corresponds to the exterior, yang brightness to the interior, and lesser yang to half-exterior and half-interior. The lesser yang stage represents an intermediate position of the pathogenic factor.

Clinical manifestations include alternating chills and fever, fullness of the costal and hypochondriac regions, a dull facial expression, loss of appetite, irritability, dry throat, nausea, a bitter taste in the mouth, blurred vision, a white, slippery tongue coating on the right side only and a wiry pulse.

The alternating chills and fever reflect the struggle between the pathogenic factor and the body's qi. It is important to distinguish this from the fever and aversion to cold associated with the greater yang stage. In the greater yang stage there is simultaneous fever and aversion to cold, while in the lesser yang stage the fever and chills alternate. The fullness in the costal and hypochondriac region is from stagnation of qi in the Gallbladder channel due to obstruction from the pathogenic factor. The dull facial expression reflects a diminishment of the lesser yang channels' ability to promote the circulation of qi. Loss of appetite is due to accumulation of interior heat in the lesser yang causing derangement of Stomach qi. The bitter taste, dry throat and blurred vision are all caused by the flaring of Gallbladder heat. The white, slippery tongue coating on the right side reflects the position of the pathogenic factor between the exterior and the interior, and the wiry pulse indicates the presence of the pathogenic factor in the Gallbladder channel. The key symptoms are alternating chills and fever, fullness in the hypochondriac region, loss of appetite and a bitter taste in the mouth.

From a biomedical perspective, diseases including influenza, mononucleosis (glandular fever), ear infections and malaria may present with this pattern. It is very common in certain influenza-like viral infections such as myalgic encephalomyelitis (chronic fatigue syndrome) that drag on for weeks or months with chills and fever.

GREATER YIN

The greater yin stage marks the penetration of the pathogenic factor to deeper energetic layers affecting the yin Organs. In the three yang stages only the yang Organs or channels are affected. The three yin stages are generally, but not exclusively, characterized by deficiency and cold.

The greater yin stage involves invasion of the middle burner (Spleen) by cold as well as Spleen deficiency. Clinical manifestations include abdominal fullness, vomiting, loss of appetite, diarrhea, absence of thirst, a pale tongue body and white tongue coating and a deep, slow pulse.

This stage is caused by direct invasion of cold attacking the Spleen when the Spleen yang is deficient. Spleen yang deficiency impairs the transforming and transporting functions of this Organ, which in turn causes abdominal fullness, vomiting, diarrhea and loss of appetite. The abdominal discomfort is somewhat relieved by pressure. The absence of thirst reflects the cold pattern, which is also indicated by the pale tongue and slow pulse.

From a biomedical perspective, diseases such as viral infections affecting the digestive tract may present with this pattern.

LESSER YIN

The lesser yin stage is also an interior pattern affecting the yin Organs, especially the Heart and Kidneys. There are two patterns within the lesser yin stage: transformation to cold (or lesser yin cold), and transformation to heat (lesser yin heat).

Lesser Yin Cold

Clinical manifestations of lesser yin cold include chills, aversion to cold, listlessness and sleepiness, cold limbs, diarrhea containing undigested food particles, absence of thirst or a desire to drink warm fluids, profuse, clear urine, a pale tongue body and a deep, thin pulse. In this stage the patient tends to lie in a curled-up position.

The aversion to cold, coldness of the limbs, listlessness and curled-up position of the body when lying down are all symptoms associated with yang deficiency. The whole pattern is basically due to Kidney yang deficiency which, for example, affects the Spleen yang and causes diarrhea. The profuse, clear urine reflects the internal cold and the deep, thin pulse denotes the condition of interior deficiency.

Lesser Yin Heat

Clinical manifestations of lesser yin heat include fever, irritability, insomnia, dryness of the mouth and throat, scanty, yellow urine, a red tongue without coating and a thin, rapid pulse.

This stage is characterized by yin deficiency of the Kidneys. Fever and dryness of the mouth and throat are caused by Kidney yin deficiency, as are irritability and insomnia. The latter symptoms are the result of Kidney yin deficiency causing deficiency heat of the Heart, which in turn causes the spirit to suffer. The scanty, yellow urine, red tongue and rapid pulse are caused by deficiency heat burning the body fluids.

TERMINAL YIN

Although the terminal yin stage may correspond to problems in the Pericardium and Liver, it may also involve other pathologies. It is a pattern of mixed heat and cold and includes disorders caused by parasites. Clinical manifestations include persistent thirst, a feeling of energy rising to the chest, pain and a sensation of heat in the chest, a feeling of hunger with no desire to eat, cold limbs, diarrhea and vomiting (including the vomiting of roundworms).

The persistent thirst is due to Liver heat consuming the body fluids. The feeling of energy rising to the chest and the hot, painful sensations in the chest are caused by the rising of Liver heat. Hunger with no desire to eat, vomiting and diarrhea are caused by Liver heat and the retention of cold in the Intestines and Stomach. Liver heat makes the patient hungry, but the cold in the Stomach and Intestines suppresses the patient's desire to eat. The vomiting of roundworms is due to cold in the Intestines to which the worms cannot adapt. There is a separation of yin and yang energies with the yang rising to the top of the body away from the limbs, hence the coldness in the limbs.

In summary, this pattern is characterized by a set of concurrent deficiency cold and excess heat signs. The signs of deficiency cold include the absence of a desire to eat, vomiting, diarrhea and coldness of the limbs. The excess heat signs are persistent thirst, pain in the chest, a feeling of energy rising to the chest and hunger.

II
Identification of Patterns According to the Four Levels

INTRODUCTION

The identification of patterns according to the four levels is concerned with febrile diseases caused by externally-contracted heat. It was developed by Wu You-Ke, Ye Tian-Shi and Wu Ju-Tong during the early Qing dynasty, although elements of its conceptualization of the disease process can be found in the *Inner Classic* and the *Discussion of Cold-induced Disorders*.

Ye Tian-Shi, the main representative of the School of Warm Diseases *(wēn bìng)*, was born in 1667 in the city of Suzhou. He died in 1746. This was a time when infectious diseases were widespread in China, diseases which from the perspective of Chinese medicine are derived from externally-contracted heat. Ye Tian-Shi was the most famous doctor of the early Qing dynasty. He wrote several books, among which the *Discussion of Warm-Febrile Diseases*[1] and the *Clinical Guide of Case Histories*[2] are the most prominent. In addition to being an authority on diseases from externally-contracted heat and developing the identification of patterns according to the four levels, Ye Tian-Shi was also a specialist in the treatment of measles and of children's diseases in general. Another of his books is entitled *Essentials of Pediatrics*.[3]

The identification of patterns according to the four levels is devoted exclusively to warm-febrile diseases, i.e., those caused by externally-contracted heat. These types of diseases are characterized by the following aspects:

- They are always caused by exterior heat or wind-heat.
- They always display fever as a main symptom.
- The heat is intense and has a strong tendency to burn the body fluids and injure yin.

- They are contagious.
- The pathogenic factor penetrates via nose and mouth.

There are also febrile diseases caused by cold, the analysis of which is based upon the six-stage identification of patterns discussed in Appendix I.

The essence of the four-level identification of patterns is the concept of four energetic layers in the body. These four layers, or levels, are each associated with a particular type of energy and are called the defensive-qi *(wèi)*, qi *(qì)*, nutritive qi *(yíng)* and blood *(xuè)* levels. In order of depth, defensive-qi is the most superficial, and blood the deepest level. In this system each energetic level is characterized by a detailed pattern of symptoms. Once the physician has identified the energetic level at which the disease resides, an appropriate treatment is applied.

Even though this system of differentiation was designed for externally-contracted diseases, it can also be applied in cases of internally-generated diseases from heat, since the heat becomes internalized once it penetrates the defensive-qi and qi levels.

DEFENSIVE-QI LEVEL

The defensive-qi level includes four possible patterns: wind-heat, summer-heat, damp-heat and dry-heat. These four patterns present with different clinical manifestations but, in the initial stages, they all display signs and symptoms of invasion of the exterior by wind-heat. The following description of clinical manifestations will therefore be based mostly on the signs and symptoms of invasion by wind-heat.

The defensive-qi level is the most superficial level of attack by external heat, a stage at which the signs and symptoms are manifested at the defensive-qi energetic level. This corresponds to the greater yang stage of the six-stage identification of patterns, except that here the pathogenic factor is heat rather than cold. The defensive-qi level is characterized by impairment of defensive qi energy. The four principal functions of the defensive qi are resisting external pathogenic factors; warming and nourishing the skin and muscles; controlling the skin, hair and the opening and closing of the pores; and connecting with the Lung qi. In the defensive-qi level all of these functions are impaired, which gives rise to specific clinical manifestations.

Signs and symptoms of the defensive-qi level include fever, slight shivers, aversion to cold or wind, absence of or only slight sweating, headache, cough, sore throat, thirst, a tongue body that is slightly red on the tip and/or edges, a thin, white tongue coating and a floating, rapid pulse.

The fever associated with this stage is due to the struggle between the external pathogenic heat and the defensive qi. Aversion to cold or wind is caused by the impairment of the defensive qi's function of warming and nourishing the skin and muscles. Absence of or only slight sweating is due to a decline in the defensive qi's function of regulating the opening and closing of the pores. Headache (primarily occipital) is due to obstruction of the circulation of defensive qi. The cough is due to obstruction of the defensive qi, which impairs the Lungs' descending function. The sore throat is caused by the heat in the Lung channel, and thirst by heat drying the body fluids. The slightly red tip and/or edges of the tongue reflect the invasion of the exterior energetic layers by heat. The floating pulse reflects the struggle of the defensive qi with the external pathogenic factor; the rapid nature of that pulse also reflects the presence of heat.

From a biomedical perspective, diseases including upper respiratory tract infections, tonsillitis, the initial stages of German measles, chicken pox and measles may present with this pattern.

QI LEVEL

The qi level is the second level in the invasion of external heat. In the defensive-qi level, the clinical manifestations actually reflect an impairment of the defensive qi. In the qi level, the word "qi" does not imply any particular type of qi; rather, it serves to indicate a further penetration of the external heat to a level that is still not too deep. Basically, the qi level indicates two things: first, that the body's resistance is still good; and second, that the normal functioning of the Organs is impaired, though not profoundly, by the pathogenic factor.

There are five conditions associated with the qi stage: heat in the chest and diaphragm, heat in the Stomach channel, dry heat in the Intestines, Stomach and Spleen damp-heat, and heat in the Gallbladder channel.

Heat in the Chest and Diaphragm

Clinical manifestations of heat in the chest and diaphragm include fever, no aversion to cold, a feeling of heat, breathlessness, a cough with yellow or rusty-colored and purulent sputum, a distressing, burning sensation in the epigastrium, thirst, a slippery, rapid pulse and a red tongue with a thick yellow coating (PLATE 41).

Most of these clinical manifestations reflect the accumulation of externally-contracted heat in the chest and diaphragm, causing obstruction of qi in this area. The fever is not high. The yellow tongue coating reflects a deeper penetration of the disease than in the defensive-qi level; however, it is only light yellow and could also be partly white. The thirst is caused by heat drying the body fluids. The productive cough is caused by the impairment of the Lung descending function by heat.

From a biomedical perspective, diseases including acute bronchitis, pneumonia and lung abscess may present with this pattern.

Heat in the Stomach Channel

Clinical manifestations of heat in the Stomach channel include high fever, no aversion to cold, profuse sweating, aversion to heat, thirst, a red tongue with a dry-yellow coating and a rapid, overflowing pulse.

In this pattern the heat is severe, but the body's qi is also strong. The high fever reflects the struggle between the external heat and the body's qi. Sweating is due to heat steaming in the interior, and is profuse. Thirst and the yellow, dry tongue coating are caused by heat consuming the body fluids. The thirst is severe and the patient craves cold water. The overflowing and rapid pulse reflects the presence of heat in the interior. This pattern is identical to the yang brightness channel stage of the six-stage identification of patterns described in Appendix I.

From a biomedical perspective, diseases including influenza, pneumonia and encephalitis may present with this pattern.

Dry Heat in the Intestines

Clinical manifestations of dry heat in the Intestines include high fever in the afternoon, constipation, a burning sensation in the anus, abdominal distension, fullness and pain which is worse on pressure, irritability, a faint feeling, a red tongue with a thick, very dry yellow, brown or black coating and a deep, full and rapid pulse.

This pattern is practically the same as the yang brightness Organ pattern of the six stages. It is characterized by extreme heat in the Intestines desiccating feces and causing constipation and abdominal pain. This corresponds to fire — as opposed to heat — and is described in chapter 8. Fire dries up the fluids more than does heat, hence the constipation and the very dry tongue coating. Fire also disturbs the spirit more, hence the pronounced irritability or even delirium. The deep, full pulse reflects the deeper position of fire compared to that of heat.

From a biomedical perspective, this pattern may be seen in febrile intestinal infections.

Stomach and Spleen Damp-Heat

The clinical manifestations of this pattern include a continuous fever which does not abate with sweating, a feeling of heaviness of the body and head, a feeling of oppression of the chest and abdomen, nausea, loose stools, a sticky-yellow tongue coating and a slippery, rapid pulse.

All of these manifestations reflect the obstruction of the middle and lower burner by dampness and heat. In particular, the slippery, greasy or sticky coating is typical of dampness.

From a biomedical perspective, this pattern may be seen in febrile intestinal infections, food poisoning or gastroenteritis.

Heat in the Gallbladder Channel

Clinical manifestations of heat in the Gallbladder channel include alternating hot and cold feeling (with hot predominating), a bitter taste in the mouth, thirst, a dry throat, hypochondriac pain, fullness in the epigastrium, nausea, a yellow, sticky tongue coating on one side and a wiry, rapid pulse.

This pattern is similar to the lesser yang stage of the six-stage identification of patterns, except that there is dampness and more heat than cold. Likewise, the analysis of the clinical manifestations is the same as that of the lesser yang stage, except for the fullness in the epigastrium and the sticky, yellow tongue coating, which reflects dampness in the middle burner.

From a biomedical perspective, diseases including influenza, infectious mononucleosis (glandular fever), myalgic encephalomyelitis (chronic fatigue syndrome), acute cholecystitis and malaria may present with this pattern.

NUTRITIVE-QI LEVEL

Nutritive qi is that which flows through the channels and blood vessels to nourish the body. In the nutritive-qi level, the pathogenic factor has penetrated deeper to the level of the nutritive qi and the Organs are therefore affected. Because nutritive qi is closely related to blood and flows through the blood vessels, it affects the Heart and Pericardium. Some of the signs and symptoms of this level reflect the impairment of the Heart and Pericardium functions.

Clinical manifestations include feverishness that is worse at night, dryness of the mouth, absence of thirst, faint skin eruptions (maculae), irritability, insomnia, a deep red tongue body with little or no coating (PLATE 42) and a thin, rapid pulse. In severe cases there may be delirium.

Most of the symptoms are caused by the burning up of the yin. Fever at night is due to insufficiency of yin qi. The dry mouth is related to a diminishment of body fluids due to heat, but there is no thirst because the diminishment in body fluids is not too severe. The skin eruptions are caused by heat in the blood vessels. Irritability, insomnia and possibly delirium all arise from heat affecting the Heart and therefore the spirit. The red tongue without coating and the thin, rapid pulse are due to insufficiency of yin.

From a biomedical perspective, diseases including encephalitis, meningitis and lobar pneumonia may present with this pattern.

BLOOD LEVEL

The blood level is the last and deepest level of heat's penetration into the body, with the most serious manifestations. The word "blood" in this context merely denotes a deeper energetic layer, since the nutritive qi and blood are closely connected and are indeed inseparable.

Clinical manifestations include high fever, skin that is hot to the touch, skin eruptions (maculae) of a purple or black color, epistaxis, hemoptysis, bloody stool, manic behavior, a deep red tongue body without coating and a thin, rapid pulse. In severe cases there may be delirium. Most of the signs and signs, such as the skin eruptions and the various hemorrhages, are due to heat in the blood. The manic behavior and delirium are caused by heat stirring the blood and affecting the Heart (which governs blood) and the spirit.

From a biomedical perspective, diseases including encephalitis, meningitis and acute leukemia may present with this pattern.

NOTES

1. Ye Tian-Shi, *Discussion of Warm-febrile Diseases (Wen re lun)* (mid-18th century).

2. Ye Tian-Shi, *Clinical Guide of Case Histories (Ling zheng zhi nan yin an)* (1766).

3. Ye Tian-Shi, *Essentials of Pediatrics (You ke yao lue)* (mid-18th century).

III
Identification of Patterns According to the Three Burners

INTRODUCTION

This system of differentiation, like the four-level identification of patterns, is concerned with febrile diseases caused by externally-contracted heat. It was developed by Wu Ju-Tong (1758-1836), a native of Jiangsu Province. During Dr. Wu's lifetime there was a continuing prevalence of infectious febrile diseases such as measles, scarlet fever and smallpox, and it was therefore natural that the medical specialist's attention was concentrated on the study of these diseases.

The differentiation of diseases according to the three burners is set forth in Wu's book, *A Systematic Differentiation of Febrile Diseases*. Although no new pattern is presented in his work, he explained and developed the theory of warm-febrile diseases as formulated by previous physicians, notably Ye Tian-Shi (APPENDIX II). Dr. Wu's work therefore represents an important systematization of all the previous theories concerning warm-febrile diseases.

The concept of the three burners involves a three-fold division of the body into upper, middle and lower burners. The upper burner encompasses that part of the body from the top of the head to the diaphragm. The middle burner consists of the area from the diaphragm to the umbilicus. The lower burner extends from the umbilicus to the feet.

This three-fold division, however, is more often used in relation to the trunk of the body alone. In this context, the upper burner consists of the area from the throat to the diaphragm, corresponding to the Heart/Pericardium and Lungs. The middle burner encompasses the area from the diaphragm to the umbilicus, corresponding to the Stomach and Spleen. The lower burner extends from the umbilicus to (and including) the external genitalia, corresponding to the Liver, Kidneys, Bladder, Intestines and, in women, the Womb.

The identification of patterns according to the three burners classifies clinical manifestations based upon their location in either the upper, middle or lower burner. This scheme is applied in cases of attack by external heat and is used in conjunction with the four-level identification of patterns (APPENDIX II). The difference is that whereas the four-level identification of patterns distinguishes the depth of penetration of pathogenic heat in terms of severity, the three-burner differentiation identifies the level, in vertical terms on the body, to which the heat has penetrated.

UPPER BURNER

The Organs of the upper burner are the Lungs and Heart, and the clinical manifestations of disease in this stage correspond to those of an attack of heat on these Organs. However, in Chinese medicine it is thought that the Heart cannot be invaded by external pathogenic factors; the clinical manifestations are therefore those of invasion of the Pericardium by heat.

Lungs

Invasion of the Lungs by external wind-heat may be manifested at the most superficial level (defensive-qi level) or more deeply in the Lungs themselves. This distinction is based upon analysis of the symptoms according to the four-level differentiation, so that, within the upper burner patterns, there is invasion of the Lung's defensive-qi portion by wind-heat and heat in the Lungs (at the qi level).

The clinical manifestations of invasion of the Lungs at the defensive-qi level are identical to those of the defensive-qi level of the four-level differentiation.

The signs and symptoms of invasion of the Lungs themselves are feverishness, sweating, cough, wheezing, thirst with a desire to drink, a feeling of oppression and pain in the chest, a red tongue body with yellow coating and a rapid pulse. These manifestations are virtually the same as those of "heat in the chest and diaphragm" of the qi level within the four-level identification of patterns.

The fever and sweating are due to heat steaming in the Lungs. The feeling of oppression and pain in the chest, cough and wheezing are caused by impairment of the Lungs' descending function due to the pathogenic heat. The thirst with desire to drink is related to consumption of body fluids by heat. Similarly, the red tongue body, yellow coating and rapid pulse all reflect the presence of heat.

From a biomedical perspective, diseases including acute bronchitis, pneumonia and encephalitis may present with this pattern.

Pericardium

An invasion of the Pericardium by pathogenic heat can develop from the invasion of the Lungs by heat, or from the defensive-qi level pattern of the four-level differentiation. If it develops from one of these patterns it represents a worsening of the condition, and usually occurs with a sudden change in the condition.

Clinical manifestations include feverishness, a burning sensation in the epigastrium, coldness of the limbs, delirium, aphasia, difficulty in moving the tongue, and a deep red tongue body with red points on the tip without coating.

The feverishness and cold limbs are caused by heat being confined in the interior, unable to reach the extremities. The deeper the confinement of the heat, the colder the limbs. The delirium and aphasia are due to heat consuming the body fluids and transforming into phlegm, blurring the Heart and spirit and rendering the Heart unable to move the tongue. The deep red tongue without coating is associated with heat at the nutritive-qi level.

From a biomedical perspective, diseases including heatstroke, meningitis and encephalitis may present with this pattern.

MIDDLE BURNER

An invasion of the middle burner by pathogenic heat involves two patterns: heat in the yang brightness and damp-heat in the Spleen. Heat in the yang brightness is identical to the yang brightness Organ pattern of the six-stage identification of patterns. Invasion of the Spleen by damp-heat is seen in the early stages of diseases caused by externally-contracted heat and is the same as the pattern "Stomach and Spleen damp-heat" at the qi level of the four-level identification of patterns.

Clinical manifestations include aversion to cold, slight feverishness that worsens in the afternoon, a heavy sensation in the head, as if it were wrapped in a bag, a heavy sensation throughout the body and limbs, fullness of the chest and epigastrium, nausea and vomiting, a white, sticky tongue coating and a weak, floating and rapid pulse.

The aversion to cold is caused by obstruction of the yang qi by damp-heat. The slight feverishness is due to damp-heat, with the dampness more predominant than the heat. The heavy sensation in the head is due to dampness obstructing the rise of yang qi to the head. The heavy sensation in the body and limbs is due to dampness obstructing and impairing the Spleen's transporting and transformative functions, such that the flow of qi is retarded in the muscles (controlled by the Spleen). The feeling of fullness in the chest and epigastrium is caused by obstruction of the middle burner by dampness and heat, which interferes with the ascending and descending of qi in the middle burner. The sticky tongue coating and weak, floating pulse reflect the presence of dampness.

From a biomedical perspective, diseases including infectious mononucleosis, influenza and enteritis may present with this pattern.

LOWER BURNER

Heat in the lower burner attacks the Kidneys or the Liver.

Kidneys

When heat invades the Kidneys it dries up the Kidney yin and leads to heat from deficiency. Clinical manifestations include a slight, lingering fever, hot palms and soles, dryness of the mouth, lassitude, deafness, a red, peeled tongue and a thin, rapid or a floating, empty pulse.

The heat in the palms and soles, low-grade fever and dry mouth are all caused by heat from yin deficiency drying up the body fluids. The deafness is due to weakness of the Kidney yin, which is unable to reach the ears. The red, peeled tongue and thin, rapid pulse reflect deficiency heat.

Liver

Although the Liver is anatomically located in the middle burner, it is placed in the lower burner due to its close functional relationship with the Kidneys. The Liver pattern is characterized by heat giving rise to Liver wind. It can evolve from the Kidney pattern when heat has exhausted the yin.

Clinical manifestations include low-grade fever, coldness of the limbs, dry, black teeth, drying and cracking of the lips, convulsions and trembling, a dry, reddish-purple tongue body and a deep, thin and rapid pulse.

The low-grade fever is caused by heat injuring the yin. The cold limbs are due to consumption of the Kidney yin by heat and the separaVtion of the yin and yang, such that the two cannot communicate. The yin is consumed and the yang does not circulate. The black, dry teeth, dry lips and thin, rapid pulse are caused by yin deficiency with deficiency heat. The convulsions and tremors are due to Liver wind, which arises from the consumption of the Kidney and Liver yin by heat.

From a biomedical perspective, diseases including encephalitis and meningitis may present with this pattern.

IV
Summary of Tongue Signs in Externally-contracted Cold or Heat

TABLE 1.
DIFFERENTIATION OF PATTERNS ACCORDING TO THE SIX STAGES

The main point to remember is that in the three yang stages the body color is generally unchanged and that changes of the coating are of primary importance, while in the three yin stages the changes of the tongue body are of primary importance.

PATTERN	TONGUE BODY	TONGUE COATING
Greater yang	Unchanged	Thin and white, possibly more around the center or in the front third
Yang brightness	Red	Yellow, thick and dry
Lesser yang	Unchanged	White and slippery on one side only, or white and gray or white and black
Greater yin	Pale	White
Lesser yin Cold Heat	 Pale Red	 White No coating
Terminal yin	Pale	White and yellow (because of both heat and cold signs)

TABLE 2.
IDENTIFICATION OF PATTERNS
ACCORDING TO THE FOUR LEVELS

PATTERN	TONGUE BODY	TONGUE COATING
Defensive-qi level	Slightly red on front and/or edges	Thin, white
Qi level	Red or normal	Yellow
Nutritive-qi level	Deep red	No coating
Blood level	Deep red or reddish purple	No coating

TABLE 3.
IDENTIFICATION OF PATTERNS
ACCORDING TO THE THREE BURNERS

PATTERN	TONGUE BODY	TONGUE COATING
Upper Burner:		
Wind-heat in Lungs	Slightly red on front and/or edges	Yellow
Lung heat	Red	Yellow
Pericardium heat	Deep red, red points	No coating
Middle Burner:		
Heat in yang brightness	Red	Yellow, dry
Damp-heat in Spleen	Red	Sticky, yellow
Lower Burner:		
Kidneys	Deep red	No coating
Liver	Deep red	No coating

V
Tongues Signifying Dangerous Conditions

Certain tongues denote particularly serious conditions and are usually regarded as signifying imminent death if they appear suddenly in the course of an acute disease. Under other circumstances they may persist for several years before the patient dies. These "dangerous tongues" are usually taken to mean the collapse of yin or yang. Such a collapse involves a state of extreme and serious deficiency and even total "separation" of yin and yang. In general, any tongue without spirit can be a manifestation of a significant problem. Especially when the root has a dark, dry and withered look, the prognosis is poor.

There are a variety of conditions associated with collapse of yin. If there is no tongue coating and the tongue looks like a pig's kidney or like a mirror, this is due to heat injuring the yin or to collapse of the Stomach qi. If the tongue looks like a patch of fish scales, has prickles on its surface and is dry with withered cracks, it is caused by exhaustion of the body fluids. A white and moldy coating indicates Kidney and Stomach yin deficiency leading to heat, with damp-toxin lurking inside. This type of coating is only found in chronic conditions of long duration. Finally, when the tongue body is red in the middle and black on the sides, collapse of the Kidney yin is indicated.

Collapse of yang may also be evident from examination of the tongue. The collapse of Spleen yang is indicated when the tongue body is pale and the coating is like snow flakes. A blue tongue without coating is always a sign of danger. The blue body color indicates cold congealed inside with blood stasis, and the absence of coating signifies the total collapse of qi and blood. This is one of the rare cases in which the absence of coating is due to extreme deficiency of yang, rather than deficiency of yin.

Sometimes a tongue can signify extreme problems with either the yin or the yang depending on the rest of the presentation. A black, dry and cracked tongue usually indicates a severe, dangerous withering and exhaustion of the Kidney yin. However, in rare and extreme cases this coating can also arise from true cold in the interior with yang deficiency, even though the tongue is dry. This occurs when the yang qi cannot move and evaporate the fluids, which makes the coating dry. It is of the utmost importance to look for other signs such as the absence of thirst and scanty, clear urine so that this condition is not mistaken for a heat pattern.

A few other tongues also signify a dangerous collapse of vital body functions. If the tip of the tongue is contracted and the tongue itself is completely dry and resembles dry meat, there is exhaustion of the qi and blood. The same cause is present when the tongue is dry and red like a persimmon or tomato. A tongue body which is short like a kidney indicates collapse of the Liver qi. When the coating suddenly changes from thick to thin, it indicates the sudden collapse of Stomach qi.

Intense stasis is also a very dangerous condition that is usually observable in the tongue. A reddish purple color with a redder tip and swelling anteriorly represents blood stasis with heat and severe blood stasis in the chest. Finally, in pregnant women a blue tongue may indicate the danger of imminent miscarriage.

Glossary of Chinese Terms

斑 *bān*	spots (on tongue)
本 *běn*	root
痹 *bì*	painful obstruction
辨证 *biàn zhèng*	identification of patterns
标 *biāo*	manifestation
尺 *chí*	proximal or rear (pulse position)
刺 *cì*	thorns or prickles (on tongue)
寸 *cùn*	distal or front (pulse position)
点 *diǎn*	points (on tongue)
腑 *fǔ*	yang Organs
谷气 *gǔ qì*	food qi
关 *guān*	middle (pulse position)
後天之气 *hòu tiān zhī qì*	acquired qi
滑 *huá*	slippery
筋 *jīn*	sinews
津液 *jīn yè*	body fluids
精 *jīng*	essence
命门 *mìng mén*	gate of vitality
弄 *nòng*	moving (tongue)
强 *qiáng*	stiff (tongue)
三焦 *sān jiāao*	three burners (anatomical divisions) or Triple Burner (yang Organ)

舌苔 *shé tāi*	tongue coating
舌质 *shé zhì*	tongue body
神 *shén*	spirit
实 *shí*	excess or full
卫气 *wèi qì*	defensive qi
痿软 *wěi ruǎn*	flabby (tongue)
痿证 *wěi zhèng*	atrophy disorder
五行 *wǔ xíng*	five phases
先天之气 *xiān tiān zhī qì*	congenital qi
虚 *xū*	deficient or empty
营气 *yíng qì*	nutritive qi
原气 *yuán qì*	original qi
脏 *zàng*	yin Organs
脏腑 *zàng fǔ*	Organs or internal Organs
证 *zhèng*	pattern or disorder
中风 *zhòng fēng*	wind-stroke or attack of wind
中气 *zhōng qì*	middle qi
肿胀 *zhǒng zhàng*	swollen (tongue)

Select Bibliography

CLASSICAL TEXTS

1. *Classic of the Spiritual Axis (Ling Shu Jing)*灵枢经. Beijing: People's Medical Publishing House, 1963.

2. *Classic of Difficulties with Explanations (Nan Jing Yi Shi)*难经译释. Edited by the Classics Research and Teaching Group of the Nanjing College of Traditional Chinese Medicine. Shanghai: Shanghai Scientific Publishing House, 6th edition, 1980.

3. *Classic of Difficulties with Annotations (Nan Jing Jiao Shi)*难经校释. Edited by Nanjing College of Traditional Chinese Medicine. Beijing: People's Medical Publishing House, 1979.

4. *Discussion of Cold-induced Disorders with Explanations (Shang Han Lun Yi Shi)*伤寒论译释. Edited by the Cold-induced Diseases Research and Teaching Group of the Nanjing College of Traditional Chinese Medicine. Shanghai: Shanghai Scientific Publishing House, 1980.

5. *Essentials of the Golden Cabinet: A New Explanation (Jin Gui Yao Lue Xin Jie)* 金匮要略新解. Edited by He Ren. Zhejiang: Zhejiang Scientific Publishing House, 1981.

6. *Yellow Emperor's Inner Classic: Simple Questions (Huang Di Nei Jing Su Wen)* 黄帝内经素问. Beijing: People's Medical Publishing House, 1963.

MODERN TEXTS

1. Academy of Traditional Chinese Medicine. *A Concise Dictionary of Chinese Medicine (Jian Ming Zhong Yi Ci Dian)*简明中医辞典. Beijing: People's Medical Publishing House, 2nd edition, 1980.

2. Beijing College of Traditional Chinese Medicine. *Practical Chinese Medicine (Shi Yong Zhong Yi Xue)* 实用中医学. Beijing: Beijing Publishing House, 4th edition, 1980.

3. Beijing College of Traditional Chinese Medicine. *Tongue Diagnosis in Chinese Medicine (Zhong Yi She Zhen)* 中医舌诊. Beijing: People's Medical Publishing House, 1976.

4. Guangdong College of Traditional Chinese Medicine. *Chinese Medical Diagnosis (Zhong Yi Zhen Duan Xue)* 中医诊断学. Shanghai: Shanghai Scientific Publishing House, 6th edition, 1979.

5. Jia De-Dao. *A Brief History Medicine in China (Zhong Guo Yi Xue Shi Lue)* 中国医学史略. Shanxi: Shanxi People's Publishing House, 1979.

6. Nanjing College of Traditional Chinese Medicine. *Study of Febrile Diseases (Wen Bing Xue)* 温病学. Shanghai: Shanghai Scientific Publishing House, 1978.

7. Shandong College of Traditional Chinese Medicine. *Fundamentals of Chinese Medicine (Zhong Yi Ji Chu Xue)* 中医基础学. Shandong: Shandong Scientific Publishing House, 1978.

JOURNALS

1. Academy of Traditional Chinese Medicine. *Journal of Traditional Chinese Medicine (Zhong Yi Za Zhi)* 中医杂志.

2. Chinese Medical Association. *Chinese Journal of Medical History (Zhong Hua Yi Shi Za Zhi)* 中华医史杂志.

ENGLISH LANGUAGE SOURCES

1. Lu Gwei-Djen and Needham, Joseph. *Celestial Lancets.* Cambridge: Cambridge University Press, 1980.

2. McNeil, W.H. *Plagues and Peoples.* New York: Penguin Books, 1976.

3. Shanghai College of Traditional Medicine. *Acupuncture, A Comprehensive Text.* Translated by O'Connor and Bensky. Chicago: Eastland Press, 1981.

Index